"Writer and broadcaster Glenn Deir takes us on a personal health journey that begins — as many often do — with the discovery of a lump. Writing with brutal, laser-like honesty and rare humour, Deir takes us from Japan to Newfoundland to the famed Princess Margaret Hospital in Toronto, to that dark place where we're forced to contemplate our mortality. And to that place where we surrender control of our bodies and make that leap of faith to trust our healers. This is 'medicine, from Deir's side of the gurney.' If you've ever entertained a doubt that your doctors actually know what they're doing, this is the book for you."

— Dr. Brian Goldman, host of CBC's *White Coat/Black Art* and author of *The Night Shift*.

sick j●ke

Cancer, Japan and Back Again
A Memoir

GLENN DEIR

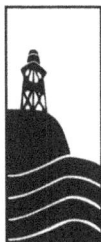

BREAKWATER BOOKS LTD.
www.breakwaterbooks.com

LIBRARY AND ARCHIVES CANADA CATALOGUING IN PUBLICATION
Deir, Glenn, 1958-
Sick joke : cancer, Japan and back again / Glenn Deir.
ISBN 978-1-55081-332-6
1. Deir, Glenn, 1958-. 2. Tonsils--Cancer--Patients--Canada--
Biography. 3. Cancer--Humor. 4. Japan--Biography. 5. Japan--
Humor. I. Title.
RC280.T7D44 2010   616.99'4320092   C2010-905945-X

© 2010 Glenn Deir
Cover Design: Rhonda Molloy
Layout: Alison Carr

We acknowledge the support of the Canada Council for the Arts which last year invested $1.3 million in the arts in Newfoundland. We acknowledge the financial support of the Government of Canada through the Canada Book Fund for our publishing activities. We acknowledge the financial support of the Government of Newfoundland and Labrador through the department of Tourism, Culture and Recreation for our publishing activities.

PRINTED IN CANADA

Canada Council   Conseil des Arts   Canada   Newfoundland
for the Arts   du Canada   Labrador

For Deb

What doesn't kill you gives you a good story.

Preface

One evening, while I was writing this book, my wife poked her head into the office and issued a stern warning.

"I'd better not be in there."

I have a confession to make. She is in here, quite a bit actually, despite her admonition. I raise the matter because she's far more private than I am and not entirely comfortable with all that I've written. But I couldn't tell the stories without transgressing on her privacy. For that, I owe her an apology. For her support, I owe her my gratitude.

"Are we still married?" I asked after she had read the finished manuscript.

"For now," she curtly replied.

I took that as a ringing endorsement and skulked away to find a publisher. Fortunately, Breakwater Books seems to have had no qualms about putting our lives on public display.

This is a book of memories. As a television reporter, I'm reminded daily of the flaws of memory. What I think is on videotape isn't there sometimes. Events and comments didn't happen exactly the way I remember them. The stories in this memoir are based on notes made shortly after the events described. Others in the book may remember the same events quite differently. Their version is equally valid.

Three of my doctors, Dr. Boyd Lee, Dr. Alia Norman and

Dr. John Waldron, kindly reviewed the book for medical mistakes; perhaps because they're decent people and they didn't want me to get it wrong, and perhaps to see whether they should sic their lawyers on me. No lawyer has called yet.

The book is medically accurate, but only for me. Don't take it as medical gospel. I'm not a doctor; I've only interviewed one on TV.

Half this book is about cancer, my cancer — the wonderfully peculiar tonsil cancer. The other half is about Japan, my Japan — the wonderfully exotic Japan. It's a tale of two journeys. Along the way, I found plenty to laugh at.

Sayonara

It began with the long gentle stroke of a razor in a far off land.

"Kole wa nan desu ka?" I said to myself.

In my stubborn effort to master conversational Japanese, I practiced whenever a situation allowed me to pluck a stock phrase from my limited repertoire. And if that meant impressing an audience of just one — namely me — so be it. Translation: *What is that?*

Actually, what I wanted to say in Japanese was "What the hell is that?" Unfortunately, I didn't know the phrase.

My Japanese teachers, being Japanese, were always polite. I had learned only courteous Japanese. The word *hell* was not part of my vocabulary. In fact, no swear word was part of my vocabulary. I wasn't even sure the Japanese had obscenities. I was Glenn the Mannerly Gaijin, the foreigner who couldn't utter a Japanese profanity even when he wanted to.

I laid the razor on the sink and ran my index finger down the left side of my neck. Caress after caress. Was I imagining it, or was there really something there? A lump? When I washed away the shaving foam I thought I could see it. Just a wee bulge. The more I stared in the mirror, the more convinced I was that it was real. There *was* a bump on my neck. Whatever it was, it felt deep. It seemed as though I could push it around slightly. It was the size of a pea.

Decision number one: say nothing to Deb. Deb Youden, the woman who had been kicking me underneath the table for almost twenty-six years in a futile effort to save me from myself.

I met Deb in Dildo. Snicker if you must, but there is such a town in Trinity Bay, Newfoundland. Not surprisingly, the road sign outside of town is its most famous attraction. Deb was the home economics teacher at the local high school. I was an ambitious, self-absorbed, and occasionally insensitive television reporter. The kind of attributes that have encouraged friends and family to add the adjective "long-suffering" to the phrase "Glenn's wife."

Deb was dozing in the bedroom of our Tokyo apartment. Why worry her unnecessarily? This lump might disappear in a day or two. Besides, the word lump would mean only one thing to her. Cancer!

Only four months earlier, Deb's younger sister had been diagnosed with non-Hodgkin's lymphoma, which is cancer of the immune system. Linda's cancer was well advanced and she was in a fight for her life. Her only hope was chemotherapy treatment.

Linda had several symptoms before the diagnosis: night sweats, chronic fatigue, abdominal pain, but what really tipped her off were the lumps that she felt around her groin, under her arms and on her neck. The lumps were swollen lymph nodes. A lump in *my* neck and Deb would surely jump to the conclusion that I had lymphoma too.

Truth was, the thought had crossed my mind even before I left the bathroom. Because of Linda's struggle I would not dismiss this lump. I would watch it. I would be very Japanese in my approach. Precise observation of the kind that allowed the Japanese to say without doubt that the subway platform was forty-two metres away, not forty-one or forty-three. You could be sure that someone had measured the distance to within a millimetre. The smallest change in my lump would not escape my attention. If the damn thing were growing, I'd pounce.

I loved Tokyo. I knew I was going to miss it terribly. The thing I loved most about the city was its constant supply of adventures, big and small. I always had the feeling that today I would see something original, meet someone exotic or learn something new.

I lived a mere thirty-minute walk from the belly of the beast — downtown Shibuya. The district is the epitome of Japanese stereotypes. A crush of people is constantly walking beneath the JumboTrons that scream buy this cosmetic or that junk food. You might even see a dinosaur stride across the side of a high-rise, as it did in the movie *Lost in Translation*. This part of Tokyo is all neon and glitter. It's maddening and exhilarating at the same time. It's the kind of spot that makes you say, "We're not in Kansas anymore, Toto."

I worked for Nippon Hoso Kyokai — the Japan Broadcasting Corporation. I was on leave from the Canadian Broadcasting Corporation. Borrowed, so to speak, from the CBC to help NHK World with its English television newscasts. I was a re-writer, but when people asked what I did for a living I'd flippantly say, "I put words in the prime minister's mouth." If I didn't like what Junichiro Koizumi had to say, I changed it. I did that quite a bit, actually. Almost every day. I was massaging the translation for the prime minister and every other non-English speaking person who appeared on *News Today: 30 Minutes*, making sure that their English sounded natural to a native speaker's ear. In short, I fixed English.

As least that's what the Good Glenn did. The Evil Glenn probably did incalculable damage to the cause of proper English in Japan. I grew up in Newfoundland. A place with dozens of accents and its own 700-page dictionary that took twenty years of scholarly research to produce. It's an English that's not spoken anywhere else on the planet. God forgive me, but I would occasionally teach my Japanese co-workers Newfoundland English. Susumu was my prize student; he understood English idioms. What harm could there be in teaching him a few Newfoundland phrases? It's not like the emperor would ever get to hear them.

We started with "How's she goin', b'y?" I swear he had the accent perfect. Hollywood actors with language coaches can't get it, but Susumu could. B'y is boy, but it sounds like bye. It's said softly and is in no way a derogatory word. The *Dictionary of Newfoundland English* describes b'y as a frequent term of address, a marker of informality or intimacy. Still, I warned Susumu to never, ever use it around a person of colour. The risk of misunderstanding was beyond calculation. The absurdity of that phrase coming out of a Japanese mouth was a guilty pleasure and always made me smile. Susumu soon graduated to "Whaddaya at?" "My nerves are rubbed raw" and "That's shockin'." Eventually, I gave Susumu a list of phrases entitled Glenn's Survival Newfoundland English. Who knows what might grow from the seed I planted? I can't wait for future linguists to sort out that version of Japanese English.

Day one, post-lump discovery. The office banter kept me somewhat distracted, but I found myself subconsciously stroking my neck in the middle of the newsroom. I would nonchalantly pull my hand down, only to find it there again later in the shift. Standing in front of a mirror, I found it impossible not to stare.

The lump was growing. Over the next couple of weeks it went from being pea-sized to marble-sized. I was in a quandary. My two-year contract was ending. My departure from Japan was only a few weeks away. Soon I would be back in the bosom of the Canadian Medicare system. Should I wait to see a doctor until then? I felt fine. I was jogging three mornings a week, sleeping well and eating all the sushi I could manage. Should I gamble that this was not a medical emergency? No, that didn't seem sensible. It was time to tell Deb and call Dr. King.

Deb could feel and see the lump too. The sun pouring into our kitchen made it all too visible. What a waste that all this attention to my neck wasn't producing any erotic sensations. Quite the opposite. Now, two people were worried.

There was one personal rule that I never broke while in Japan: when sharp objects were pointed my way, the person doing the pointing must understand English fluently. That rule lead me to a Rastafarian-looking Japanese barber, an American dentist and Dr. Leo King. Dr. King is a physician who speaks flawless English, despite being Japanese. He learned it while attending international schools in Tokyo. I had seen him previously for NHK-sponsored annual checkups. He passed the English test and he had my confidence.

"I'm wondering if I have lymphoma," I told him. I mentioned my sister-in-law and described my symptoms. He stood behind me and drove his fingers into my armpits — the first of many doctors whose digits would probe a variety of cavities in my body with impunity. Dr. King was checking for swollen lymph nodes. There are clusters of lymph nodes in the underarms. Mine were normal.

"Perhaps it's an infection," he mused. "We'll do blood work."

The follow-up appointment brought good news. My white blood cells were exactly as they should be, there was no sign of a viral or bacterial infection, I wasn't suffering from mononucleosis, I had no inflammatory disease and my liver was perfect.

"I'm not alarmed," said Dr. King. "Lymph nodes can swell up for no apparent reason and then go away."

Dr. King said he could order more sophisticated tests like CT scans, but time was running out.

"Can I safely deal with this when I return to Canada?"

"Absolutely," he said.

I had goodbye parties to attend. It was time to inflict some damage on that perfect liver of mine.

My NHK colleague Saeki-san and his wife Reiko-san had invited us to their home for a dinner party. This was a great honour. Being invited into a Japanese home was not a common occurrence for a gaijin couple. I should explain that san is a title of respect. It means Mr., Mrs., Ms. or Miss. I always used it with my bosses. But when it came to my Japanese friends, some wanted it, some didn't. In casual settings, I thought of it as the Japanese equivalent of b'y.

I liked Saeki-san from day one. Oh, he could be too much the Japanese nationalist sometimes, especially when it came to a territorial dispute with South Korea. And to my bewilderment he admired the United States of America greatly, despite the tens of thousands of U.S. soldiers still on Japanese soil. Occasionally, he fawned over superiors and was gruff to his subordinates, but in Japan that was no crime. No, what really endeared him to me was his uncanny ability to piss people off without even trying.

It was born out of a dogged determination to get the best news story on the air now, not an hour from now. Saeki-san had no time for gossips, whiners, layabouts and prima donnas, all of whom inhabit newsrooms around the world. Sometimes he rode rough-shod over people. He was smart, prickly and dedicated. He would pull a 24-hour shift and sleep on an office cot if the story warranted. I saw myself in Saeki-san, at least the old me. But if I had lost my rough edge, it wasn't enough to be casting the first stone.

One enters a Japanese home with a quality gift and not something that's been kicking around the bottom of a closet. Protocol demands that you present the hostess with a brand name gift. We brought Morozoff chocolates. Despite the Russian-sounding name the company is based in Kobe, Japan. The bag was stamped with the phrase *Sweets with Romance*. I had no idea how prophetic that would be.

Reiko-san had laid out a splendid table: gold-rimmed plates, a linen tablecloth and Japanese serving dishes. Everyone had chopsticks, but Deb and I also had silver cutlery at our places.

"No need," I announced, making no attempt to hide my cockiness. "Debbie and I use hashi all the time."

The Japanese always fuss over foreigners who have even the most rudimentary command of chopsticks. Countless meals consumed with chopsticks had made me quite proficient. I could pick up a single kernel of rice with chopsticks and had been showered with praise during my time in Japan. So it was probably at that moment that the gods decided to teach me a lesson in humility.

I raised a piece of lotus root to my mouth. Inexplicably, my chopsticks twisted, springing the lotus root. It did several somersaults before executing a perfect belly flop in the broth on my plate. I was splattered in a dozen places. Reiko-san leapt to her feet and magically produced a box of clean wipes. She explained that Saeki-san was always staining his shirts too, so she kept the box handy.

Bored with teaching humility, the gods shifted to cruel humour. My next trick was to drop a piece of greasy mackerel on the spotless tablecloth. That was followed by a dollop of red wine as a large dribble rolled down my glass. Our hosts, of course, said nothing. The Japanese would sooner die than acknowledge that a guest is soiling their tablecloth with every mouthful of food and drink. I was afraid to ask the history of this freshly ruined heirloom. Perhaps the emperor had given it to Reiko-san's grandmother.

Despite my clumsiness, we were a merry band. Bottle after bottle of wine fuelled our conversation and laughter. Someone brought up how attractive the Canadian embassy was. Another person chimed in, "That's where Prince Takamado died playing squash." The poor fellow's heart gave out and he dropped at the Canadian ambassador's feet. I apologized on behalf of Canada, and all was forgiven.

"Saeki-san, why do you like America so much? They still occupy so much of your country."

Saeki-san paused for a moment. "When President Bush went to the Twin Towers site, he told the firemen there, 'The world will soon hear you.'"

So that was it. He admired America's boldness, resolve, strength, bluntness, and might. These were all things that he desired for Japan. Saeki-san wanted Japan to be a world power, a nation that others looked up to, not one that stayed on the fringes of global events and was seen as a follower, not a leader. He was implicitly saying America is a great nation; Japan should be one too.

Reiko-san spoke to her husband in Japanese with the sweetest tone, wearing a gorgeous smile. Susumu translated for me. I was surprised to hear that she was admonishing him, but she never lost the smile or tone. *Why didn't you bring these people home sooner? They are lovely people.*

I jokingly suggested that Saeki-san was trying to decide if he liked us. No, he protested, he had always liked us.

I said, "Suki desu."

The room went stony silent. Then, all the Japanese burst into gales of laughter, except for Saeki-san who looked slightly uncomfortable.

I thought I had said, *I like you too.* When Susumu finally got his breath he explained that I had expressed a deeper — much deeper — affection for Saeki-san than *like.* It's not every day that you get to profess burning passion for a man in front of his wife, as well as your own.

The end of the evening saw us all crammed into a narrow hallway saying our goodbyes.

"Gochisosama," I said. *Thank you for a lovely meal.*

"Do itashimashite," replied Reiko-san. *Don't mention it. You're welcome.*

We placed our hands by our sides, bowed from the waist and knocked heads. My evening as Glenn the Gaijin Oaf was complete. I needn't have worried about the lump in my neck. I was going to die of humiliation.

I kept my lump a secret from friends and co-workers for as long as I could, but Japanese paternalism would eventually pry it out of me.

The Japanese live their lives following rules and social conventions that are far more intrusive than we have in Canada. Being a gaijin, I was usually excused from the duties of Japanese society. But not when it came to my health while working for a Japanese company.

NHK scheduled annual check-ups and employees were obligated to attend. The check-ups included an x-ray, hearing test, vision test, electrocardiogram, and urine and blood samples. Guess who got the report first? Not me. NHK did. Dr. King would tell NHK Human Resources all about my health and a manager would pass along the results to me. It wasn't always a discreet process. I remember one of the bosses yelling from the far end of the hallway, "Glenn-san, I have good news for you," as he waved my medical report.

When I paid for a visit to the doctor myself, the information stayed private until I used NHK's health insurance to be reimbursed. The forms demanded full disclosure. Big brother still won in the end.

My boss translated for the human resources manager filling in the paperwork.

"Why did you go to the doctor?" asked Taka-san.

"I have a lump in my neck," I said, pointing at the spot.

Perhaps Taka-san had spent too much time in California studying television and English because he said in an Arnold Schwarzenegger accent, "Ahhh, you were worried that you have a tumour."

"It's not a tumour," I said, just like Arnie in *Kindergarten Cop*. "The doctor thinks I'm fine."

I hoped I was being completely honest, but I really didn't know.

March 2007. I glanced out the window of the Narita Express train and spied cherry blossoms — the first of the season. The pink and white flowers captivate Japan every spring. The south to north movement of the cherry blossom front is treated as big news on NHK's domestic broadcasts. An area might enjoy cherry blossoms for only a week or two. The blossoms are symbolic of the fleeting nature of beauty and life. They have been revered for centuries, though deep contemplation isn't necessarily apparent in the alcohol-soaked picnics that occur underneath the cherry blossoms.

Even without the aid of cherry blossoms, I had been rather alcohol-soaked myself in recent days. The run to the airport gave me a chance to reflect on my send-off.

My NHK sayonara party took place in a second-floor bar over a lingerie shop. As I stood outside, I said to myself, "It doesn't get any better than this."

The beer flowed, the food was endless, the big bucho (boss) spoke very kind words in English, but the highlight was the goodbye tape. The NHK World crew had put together a mock newscast, in which the shock of my impending departure from Japan had rattled world leaders. President Mahmoud Ahmadinejad shouted that the Iranian people praise my great job, while a spokeswoman for North Korea dourly declared that their Great General would confer an order on me. At least that's what the subtitles said. I can't speak to the accuracy of the translation.

Susumu's voice explained over shots of crowds and neon signs that, "Glenn was lucky to live near one of the city's busiest areas — Shinjuku. It's a 24-hour nightlife and entertainment district. And a far cry from the peace and quiet of his native Newfoundland."

The video cut to pictures of ice, rocks and penguins, and up popped the word "Newfoundland." It was devastatingly funny. The crowning moment was when the camera panned from a group of stupid-looking penguins over to a Japanese scientist clicking a hand counter. It was a masterful spoof. Not only were they making fun of me, they were making fun of themselves.

Susumu appeared on camera. "Whaddaya at, b'y? I'm going to miss ya, b'y. Glenn, as a matter of fact, suki desu."

All eyes turned to me. Here was a Japanese man, speaking Newfoundland English, telling everyone that he had the hots for me. This would take some explaining, in English. But first, I wanted to give my thank you speech in Japanese. Susumu had done the translation and helped me hone my pronunciation. Many in the room had become good friends. They deserved to hear a proper thank you in *their* native tongue, not mine.

And they were entitled to laugh at my expense. They had to humble themselves every day for two years by bringing me their English scripts for correction. Sometimes they looked embarrassed and would even apologize for their perceived English shortcomings. The least I could do this night was acknowledge my own failings, linguistic and otherwise.

"To those who endured my bad Japanese, I apologize.

"To those who suffered through my boring stories about Newfoundland, I apologize.

"To those who had to correct my English, I apologize."

With each apology, with each owabi shimasu, I bowed. The deeper the bow, the bigger the laughs.

But I had a serious message too.

"In just two years, Japan has given me a lifetime of memories. I will treasure them.

"I will miss drinking beer with friends, delicious sushi, onsens (public baths with hot spring water), and beautiful women in the beautiful nation of Japan.

"I fear that I have taken more than I have given. This is a debt that I can never repay. Thank you for everything."

Listening to it all was a beaming Okawa-san — the man who had recruited me to NHK World. He was my ex-boss, my friend, and most importantly in Japan, my sempai. The closest word we have in English is mentor, but in Japan the arrangement comes with unspoken obligations. I was expected to respect and obey my sempai, and in return my sempai would guide and protect me. Our duty to each other was much more casual than it would be if I were Japanese, but it did have some of the trappings of a traditional sempai relationship. If I had a problem, Okawa-san fixed it. When I was short an annual leave day for Christmas vacation, Okawa-san told me not to worry. He assured me that when I handed in my time-card, he would "close his eyes" to what was written on that day. He was always watching my back.

Okawa-san deserves much of the credit for my easy adjustment to life in Japan. He accompanied me while I was apartment hunting, vouched for me to prospective landlords, and when I finally did choose an apartment, instructed me as to how to behave during the all-important first meeting. I had to give the elderly landlady and her daughter a token gift to show respect and gratitude. I presented them with a small box of chocolate wafers and a miniature bottle of Iceberg Vodka, brought all the way from St. John's. They were most impressed with the vodka. That, and my big hands, according to Okawa-san. He was my trusted translator. He filled in all the paperwork and I merely signed my name. I can't imagine how I would have coped without his help.

It was Okawa-san who first warned me about Deb. Not some dark secret, but the actual name Deb. Okawa-san always referred to Deb as Debbie-san. I thought nothing of it until Okawa-san pointed out that Deb sounds very much like debu in Japanese, which, in a cruel twist of linguistic fate, means fatso. I had entered a new phase of marital challenges. I went from, "Does this dress make me look fat?" to "Does this name make me look fat?"

Then I read a newspaper article that spun the tale of a man being sent to jail for twenty-nine days for calling a woman in a bar, debu. The judge described it as an utterly despicable act. I had a problem: what to call my wife in public? I polled the instructors in my Japanese class and we conducted the Goldilocks test. I wrote the three choices on the blackboard. Deb was clearly too dangerous; Deborah was too long; but Debbie was just right. From that day forward, outside the apartment, I called Deb, Debbie. When I sometimes slipped up and said, "Deb," I'd break

GLENN DEIR

out in a cold sweat. The last thing I needed was to spend twenty-nine days in a Japanese jail for calling my wife "Fatso!"

For all this and more, I saved my deepest bow and most sincere thank you for Okawa-san. Later, I did the most un-Japanese thing I could have imagined; I gave Okawa-san a bear hug. I guess that made the dam burst. Ramrod Japanese, who previously drew the line for a public display of affection at a handshake, lined up to be hugged. I even wound up embracing people I really didn't care to embrace. It was a wonderfully awkward time. The Japanese weren't sure which way to lean or where to put their arms.

After the official sayonara party wrapped, about two dozen of us headed off to that iconic symbol of Japanese culture: the karaoke parlour. Taka-san feigned disgust.

"I hate karaoke," he said. "I hate karaoke." I could tell by the twinkle in his eye that he would have a death grip on the microphone, and the rest of us would have to pry his fingers off it.

We rented a room in the same building that Bill Murray and Scarlett Johansson crooned the night away in the movie *Lost in Translation*. The hits just kept coming, and I brought the house down with a stupendously off-key version of "We Will Rock You." The applause was thunderous.

Sunrise was not far off when we finally called it a night. As we bowed and said our goodbyes, I realized that it had been one of the best nights of my life. The memories gave me a glow and made the train ride to Narita Airport the fastest ever. We were taking the long way home. First a vacation in New Zealand, followed by a few days in Seoul, Korea, and then on to Canada.

Along the way I would occasionally touch my neck and wonder, What the hell is that?

We Are Borg

Dr. Lee was whiter than I expected. You'd think that after twenty-five years of journalism and travel I would have learned never to make assumptions about people, but I had a weak moment and assumed Dr. Lee would be Asian. I was predisposed to the bias. Growing up in Grand Falls, I knew a Dr. Lee who was a cardiologist and originally from Korea. I was good friends with his two sons. My Dr. Lee, as it turned out, was originally from Petty Harbour, a few kilometres from St. John's, and couldn't be more Caucasian.

Dr. Boyd Lee looked thirty-something. Not old enough, I thought, to be a head and neck surgeon, but he had all the right credentials and a warm smile. If it came down to choosing between a curmudgeonly veteran and a pleasant up-and-comer, I'd vote for the latter.

I had to wait only a couple of weeks to get an appointment. Given the multitude of stories floating around about people waiting six months to see specialists, this was astonishing speed. The Newfoundland medical system in the spring of 2007 had many shortages and punishing waiting lists, but when it came to head and neck surgeons, St. John's was the place to be.

Dr. Lee and I discussed my unremarkable medical history. He was intrigued by my time in Japan. I was intrigued that he was practising in Newfoundland.

"If I had your skills, I'd be somewhere hot," I said. My anti-Newfoundland funk was born out of a particularly vile spring. Freezing temperatures, howling winds, and an endless cycle of rain, drizzle and fog. It was so unlike Tokyo. I lack the gene that gives most Newfoundlanders weather amnesia at the first sunny day.

By now the lump was the size of a golf ball. I expected children on the street to point and ask, "Mommy, what's wrong with that man?" But no child ever did. In fact, no one mentioned it. People were either blind or excruciatingly polite.

"So," I asked Dr. Lee as I touched the lump, "what the hell is that?"

"We'll find out. Whatever it is, it's not supposed to be there."

Remember that childhood taunt, "Up your nose with a rubber hose." I now fully comprehend the tyranny of that particular procedure. Maybe it begins with ear, nose and throat doctors using pencils to do walrus impersonations at frat parties, but a key diagnostic tool for them is a fibre optic camera. A little squirt of anaesthetic spray and Dr. Lee started feeding the flexible tube up my left nostril.

"It helps to be a sadist in this job," he said.

Dr. Lee was hunched over the eyepiece. The camera gave him an excellent view of my upper air passages, all the way down to my larynx. I sneezed.

"See anything?"

"Nothing, it all looks healthy." He gently pulled the tube out. "I need to take a biopsy from the lump." Eek. That meant piercing the lump to send a piece to the lab.

The nurse produced a needle so large it belonged in a circus clown act.

"Is that the anaesthetic needle or the biopsy needle?"

"The biopsy needle. If I gave you an anaesthetic needle it would hurt more than this one."

The procedure was called a fine needle aspiration, and while the needle was indeed very fine, it looked long enough to go in one side of my neck and out the other. Dr. Lee's intention was to stick the needle directly into the lump and draw out fluid and cells. They would be sent to the pathology lab for analysis.

I flinched as the needle went deeper.

"Sorry. I must have hit the main nerve that runs from your neck out to your shoulder."

"Pus," said the nurse.

There are few words as perfect as pus. Squeeze putrid and us together and you've got the quintessential word to describe that yellow-white liquid found in human abscesses and sores. Dr. Lee drew a couple of vials and was done.

"It may be a branchial cleft cyst," said Dr. Lee. "Branchial comes from Greek and refers to gills."

Great, I thought, I was supposed to grow gills there.

Dr. Lee explained this might be a birth defect, that some of the tissue in my neck failed to develop normally, leaving a gap. Apparently, the body likes to fill in open spaces. A sac may have formed around liquid that drained from a sinus. Cysts are usually benign, but they are prone to infection, so surgery is the recommended treatment.

"We'll know more after we get the lab results," he said.

My return to the Canadian Broadcasting Corporation in St. John's was uneventful. After a flurry of handshakes and welcome backs, people promptly lost interest in my Japan adventure. I expected as much and wasn't deflated by it. I knew I would have to fit into their world and not the other way around. Still, no matter how much I steeled myself, reverse culture shock snuck up on me. Nothing felt right for the first few weeks, not even my house. The space seemed gratuitous and I couldn't remember where items were kept. It was as though I didn't belong.

The distance I felt between St. John's and Tokyo couldn't be measured in kilometres. I had half a heart in each city. At least I could call my wife "Deb" in public again and not worry about being thrown in jail.

Social occasions only emphasized the great divide. My sister Barb and her husband came into town for a weekend. Part of her Saturday night ritual was playing radio bingo. We all listened in the kitchen. Deb and I quietly chopped and diced, lest we drown out the bingo caller.

"The jackpot for our final game is $7200 and it will go tonight. But this is game number three for $500, and we're playing the inside box. No B's or O's in this game."

Not quite as challenging as Sudoku, but radio bingo practitioners are just as passionate. However, passion wasn't enough for my sister. Her bingo dabber was not as active as it needed to be to win.

I doubted anyone was playing radio bingo in Tokyo and I was certain no one was eating seal flipper pie. Later that week the Topsail United Church was having its annual seal flipper dinner in the church basement. Deb's dad was treating the family, including the elderly Uncle Fred and Aunt Emmie. Uncle Fred is hard of hearing; Aunt Emmie speaks whatever is on her mind, loudly. So in the middle of the Anchormen Chorus singing "My Wild Irish Rose," Aunt Emmie yelled across the table to Uncle Fred, explaining that her neighbour had a tragic and sudden demise.

"He blew his brains out."

"What?"

"HE BLEW HIS BRAINS OUT."

"Sure, I thought he never had any brains."

Heads all around the room turned toward our table. Deb was shushing the pair of them, while the barbershop quartet serenaded us about the sweetest flower that grows. We were back in Kansas again, Toto.

Dr. Lee was apologetic; he would need to take another Bozo the Clown needle and push it into my neck. The lab report from the first biopsy mentioned abnormal cells, but the doctor couldn't make a diagnosis. I offered to let the resident doctor from British Columbia who was shadowing Dr. Lee have a jab at me, but he only wanted her to watch.

The second pathology report was ready in a few days, but it was also inconclusive. The needle failed to draw enough cells for interpretation. The pathologist advised further investigation as clinically warranted. Translation: Cut the damn thing out.

"I'll let you know about scheduling," said Dr. Lee. "I'll need a second surgeon with me."

"What about the cute doctor you had last week?" I asked, my heart skipping a beat.

Dr. Lee looked dejected, dropped his head and shook it. "I never get the good-looking ones."

His mood went serious. "I need to explain what will happen if we find cancer."

Cancer. The dreaded "C" word. I thought I had left that far behind. It was a benign cyst, right? Probably, but just in case it wasn't, I needed to know the consequences. A doctor can't operate without informed consent. I was possibly facing a radical neck dissection.

Jesus, I thought, the name alone is frightening.

You are a different man after a radical neck dissection, a disfigured man. The surgeon is chasing cancer and he keeps cutting tissue until he thinks he has it all. Muscles, veins, nerves: all are potential targets.

Nerve damage could cause permanent numbness around my face, down the neck and even drop my shoulder. I might not be able to rotate my head normally and my neck would have an obvious indentation.

"You ever done this before?" I asked.

"Ya." Dr. Lee nodded with a half smile.

"I won't know any of this until I wake up, will I?"

"No, all the decisions will be made while you're asleep."

This would be major surgery under general anaesthetic. I'd

have at least a three-inch long incision, much larger if they found cancer. Now I understood why he needed a second pair of surgical hands. Dr. Lee would remove the lump and send it to the pathology lab for immediate analysis. If the pathologist spied cancer on his microscope slides, Dr. Lee and his partner would start cutting away my neck. If the lump were benign, they'd sew me up and send me off to the recovery room. I could expect to spend at least one night in hospital with a drainage tube coming out of my neck.

My God, I thought, he's going to turn me into a Borg.

Deb doesn't understand my love of *Star Trek*. I enjoy all its incarnations; I watch it whenever I can be alone with the TV. Although I'm a fan, I've never been so fanatical as to dress up as a Klingon or Romulan warrior and attend a convention. That's a little too nerdy for me. But the operation would let me be Borg for a day in the privacy of my own hospital room. I could have fun with that.

Borg are excellent villains. They are cyborg drones that maraud through the universe in cube ships, destroying worlds, assimilating millions by injecting them in the throat with nanoprobes and implanting the most hideous artificial body parts. Borg are relentless, emotionless, live as a collective, share a singular consciousness, speak of we rather than I, and always, always have tubes coming out of their necks.

Perhaps I rambled on too much about being a Borg for a day and not enough about the seriousness of the operation, because when I told Deb that I would be off work for a minimum of two weeks she was astonished.

"Two weeks! Sure, it's only minor surgery."

There are times in a marriage when a partner will grossly underestimate the severity of a situation. One can be charitable, I suppose, and calmly explain the grave circumstances and then forget about it. Or one can seize the phrase, tuck it into the back of the brain and, like a Borg, heartlessly torture a wife when she suggests in the future that events are not as serious as the husband portrays. The Evil Glenn chose the latter.

It wasn't Deb's fault that she got it wrong. Some years before when she had a cyst removed from the top of her head, she walked home from the hospital and was back to work the next day. Top of the head, side of the neck, she was thinking, what's the difference? And to be fair, perhaps I skipped over a bit. I had seen photos on the Internet of a radical neck dissection. They were sobering — an L-shaped flap of skin folded back exposing a gargantuan hole. I probably censored Dr. Lee's information the first time round.

When I broke the news about the impending operation to my sister Barb she was upset and concerned. Then to reassure me she told me that Lynn Burry, a St. John's television news anchor and a competitor, had been on the air just a couple of weeks before explaining the origin of a bright red scar down *her* neck. This was all news to me. Barb couldn't remember the details, but thankfully, Lynn was fine.

I thought, Damn it, Lynn scooped me. Not only is her newscast killing us in the ratings, she won't even let me have an exclusive story.

I was beaten before I even went under the knife.

I wondered what Mom and Dad would have thought. Their boy, raised a good Protestant, about to be operated on in a Catholic hospital. Well, it used to be Catholic. St. Clare's Mercy Hospital was solidly non-denominational when I walked through its doors; the Sisters of Mercy no longer ran the place. Still, there was a time when a black Protestant, as my Catholic friends used to call me, wouldn't be caught dead inside St. Clare's.

St. Clare's was now simply the place where the head and neck surgeons plied their trade. Deb walked alongside the wheelchair as a nurse pushed me to the operating room doors.

"You can't go any farther," she said to Deb. We kissed and hugged, and she wished me luck. I was far more relaxed than I thought I would be. And the calmness was completely natural — no happy needle for me. The prep nurses inside were jovial and chatty. One said I shouldn't worry about the scar.

"You can't see Lynn Burry's."

If I died on the table, I was going to die surrounded by NTV News viewers. There was truly no justice in the world.

Dr. Lee wandered down the hall in his hospital greens. I said, "I had a dream last night that you and the rest of the operating room staff were passing around a bottle before my operation and the assisting surgeon was three sheets to the wind."

He laughed. "It's a tradition here."

"One final thing. If you're turning me into the Borg, then I want Seven of Nine here when I wake up."

Seven of Nine. Heavy sigh. Was there ever a more sensual, well-endowed alien in a tight bodysuit? She's a bad girl gone good, a former Borg drone trying to become human again. Whenever she says, "Resistance is futile," I want to join her collective.

Dr. Lee said, "I like your style." He felt the lump and used a marker to trace the line where he would cut. "See you inside."

They didn't waste a moment once I was on the operating room table. The anaesthetist found a vein in my hand that he liked and had a quick chat with Dr. Lee on the phone about putting me to sleep. He walked behind me and that's the last thing I remember until they were calling my name in the recovery room.

Sadly, Seven of Nine wasn't hovering over me. Just a cherubic nurse saying Dr. Lee was there to see me. "That butcher," I said. He moved closer wearing a big smile.

"Was it cancer?"

"No."

"Good man."

I wasn't so much giving him credit for making the lump benign as thanking him for not gouging out my neck. He gave me a tap on the leg and said we'd talk later when I was more alert. I touched my neck just to double check that there was no deep hollow there. Everything felt normal, but I did have the promised Borg hose. It was made out of clear plastic, so the drainage from my neck turned it scarlet red. I followed the hose with my eyes to a pouch on the end. It was clipped to the bed and was small enough to fit into a shirt pocket.

I was dozy and continuously napped. Occasionally, I'd raise my knees to my chest and take ten deep breaths. A nurse had told me that would help dissipate the anaesthetic. I had no pain. I hadn't eaten since the previous evening, but food was the last thing on my mind. I sipped some water and juice.

I was wheeled upstairs to a semi-private room and a nurse washed away the brown antiseptic liquid that was smeared all over my neck and shoulder. I grabbed the buzzer when I saw Deb come in, just in case I needed to call a nurse. Deb had a history of being weak at the sight of blood or family members recovering from surgery. It helped that I felt and looked as good as I did. Deb held up rather well. No face plant or knee buckling.

She examined my scar. It ran vertically below my left ear. My neck was held together by eleven stitches. The hose was sticking out of a separate incision behind the earlobe. When I ran my index finger down my neck I could feel a flat stick underneath the skin. I was Borg all right.

Deb had chatted with Dr. Lee while I was still sleeping in the recovery room. He had already given her the good news about my being cancer-free. He also mentioned that he removed three lymph nodes. I had many questions, most of which Deb couldn't answer. I'd have to wait until Dr. Lee did his rounds.

My roommate wandered in after Deb left. He was recovering from an infected pancreas. They were pumping him with regular shots of morphine, but he was lucid enough for conversation. The biggest adjustment in his post-hospital life would be no beer.

"The doctor told me no more. But it's not like I drink. I mean, I could have a dozen beer on a Friday night and not touch any more for days. Some of the b'ys can put away a 40-ouncer, just for themselves. I only have beer. It's not like I drink."

What qualifies for drinking around dockyard workers clearly didn't match my definition of drinking.

The Venetians have a phrase, "Bed is medicine." It's so true. I felt like a new man the next day, compliments of a marathon sleep.

Dr. Lee stopped by just in the nick of time. He saved me from eating my hospital breakfast: soggy toast and a plain omelette. What more could you ask of your doctor?

I introduced Dr. Lee to my sister-in-law Karen, and after the pleasantries, he explained that the mass, my lump, was actually three lymph nodes that had matted together. They were dead and calcified, and sitting on the jugular vein. They had to be scraped off.

I thanked Dr. Lee for not drinking before the operation. He put out his hands to show that they were steady. Karen and the nurse behind Dr. Lee were obviously puzzled, if not a tad horrified, so I recounted my party in the O.R. dream. Dr. Lee said they put a little Bordeaux in the anaesthetic to make sure I passed out quickly.

He was going to send my tissue samples away for further pathology. Something in the lab report reminded him of an article he read once about a rare infection found only in Japan. Who knew? Japan — the gift that keeps on giving.

"Honto desu ka!" I exclaimed. That means *Really!*

Karen immediately blamed all the raw fish, raw horse (yes, horse, as horse was the only thing on the menu that evening), raw whale (yes, whale, despite my misgivings about the morality of Japan's "scientific" hunt) and raw chicken (yes, chicken, because everyone else was eating it) that I ate in Japan. For the record, none of them made me sick and all of them were delicious.

Karen wondered whether my body would miss the three

lymph nodes. Dr. Lee said the neck has 300 lymph nodes and I could afford to lose a few.

Dr. Lee flicked my earlobe a couple of times. "Feel that?"

"Yes."

"That's good. You might get a little tingling on your neck in the weeks ahead as the nerves re-attach."

Dr. Lee admired his handiwork. "Looks good. I don't want anyone pointing at the TV and asking, 'Who sewed that guy up?'" He explained that he cut along a fold in the skin and with time the scar would fade away. I was relieved. My only other scar is on my stomach, put there when I was a baby. It's always been noticeable. I have more finesse using a skewer on a chicken cavity than the doctor who sewed me up when I was six weeks old.

A nurse drained the pouch and measured the discharge. It was below the magic number, about two tablespoons within 24 hours.

"Send him home," said Dr. Lee.

The nurse had to remove the drainage hose. "This is going to hurt," she said. I clenched my teeth and she tugged.

"All done," she said. It hadn't hurt at all.

I looked at the end that the nurse had pulled out. It was indeed a flat stick, made of Teflon and full of tiny holes. The bulb on the other end was squeezed and that's what provided the constant suction to draw out the fluid. Ingenious!

My roommate and I were both discharged that morning. He was in pain, but was not given a prescription for painkillers. I had no pain, but *was* given a prescription for painkillers. Another of life's medical contradictions. I felt guilty, but stopped short of offering him my prescription. We exchanged only handshakes.

I went to the nursing station and bowed to the nurses behind the counter. "As we say in Japan, 'Domo arigato gozaimashita.'" *Thank you very much.*

"Whatever," said a perplexed-looking nurse.

Karen's husband picked me up. Steve had to carry my small suitcase because I was under strict orders not to lift or pull anything over five pounds. They didn't want my stitches to rip open. My immediate future would contain no housework or lawn mowing. Nothing more strenuous than picking up the TV remote control.

"I'm recovering from minor surgery" was my new buzz phrase. I used it at the first hint of a chore.

Now that I appeared destined to live, Deb wanted to kill me.

I had a coming out party of sorts a couple of weeks after my surgery. Actually, it was a friend's birthday picnic. Four couples wandering around the cliffs and beaches near Chance Cove. This movable feast had become an annual tradition and I wasn't going to let an eye-popping row of stitches stop my participation. And it was now safe for me to carry a knapsack full of wine and food.

I hadn't told our friends about my operation, so there were plenty of shocked looks and dropped jaws. I assured everyone that I was fine. Bad move. Their concern evaporated and suddenly my "friends" were calling me Frankenstein.

Our first picnic stop was a grassy meadow high atop a point of land jutting out into the North Atlantic. The wind was howling. If we hadn't nailed the tarp to the ground with our derrieres it would have flown to Ireland. Perhaps I grumbled once too often about the bloody hurricane-force winds instead of admiring the blue skies.

"Being married to you," said Deb, "is like being married to the Complaints Department."

She got a huge laugh. My 'It's only minor surgery' story was tossed aside and forgotten. The rabbles had the day's put-down and Complaints Department was it.

No one called me Frankenstein at work, at least not to my face. The three-inch red scar was impossible to ignore and eyes did stare at it, but no one asked what happened. The Evil Glenn was having a bit of sport with the shock. I think they were all under the impression that I had been away having another part of my anatomy fixed.

When I phoned my boss to inform her about my return date, she said she hoped that I would come back refreshed. I reminded her that I was on sick leave, not vacation. She made a little joke about how men and women have their own unique medical problems. I didn't set her straight, but she may have thought that I was having a vasectomy. If that was the rumour going around work, I guess I suddenly acquired a reputation for having the most unusual birth defect since Linda Lovelace in *Deep Throat*.

I bolted upright in bed when I heard the news on the radio. July 16, 2007. A strong earthquake had hit central Japan, killing at least seven people, injuring hundreds more and causing a fire in a nuclear power plant. I was relieved to hear that Tokyo had been spared. The earthquake's epicentre was over a hundred miles to the northeast. My friends were safe.

When I first came home people always asked if I had experienced an earthquake.

"One!" I'd exclaim. "I wish." I had lost count of how many times the earth shook during my two years in Japan.

I felt my first earthquake in a "mansion." An NHK colleague, Murakami-san, had invited me to join his family and friends at a fireworks show. The day was perfect: a clear sky and warm temperatures. We all met at Murakami-san's home in the afternoon.

"A very impressive mansion you have here."

"Yes, we are very rich," said a smirking Murkami-san. Mansion, or manshon, as the Japanese spell it, is their word for condominium. Murikami-san's English was good enough to understand a joke, and make one.

I played peek-a-boo with his baby girl. His older daughters proudly showed off their yukata, which are colourful cotton outfits that resemble kimono. The girls were adorable. We were sitting around the dining room table drinking iced tea and admiring the view from twenty-eight floors up. That's when the earthquake hit. There was no warning; there never is. It was as though a fist had punched us. The wallop made the tea slosh around our glasses.

It was a very strong quake. Even my Japanese friends, who have spent a lifetime on the most earthquake prone bit of real estate on the planet, looked concerned. The smack was followed by tremors, lasting about fifteen seconds. They were scary enough, but what was even more unnerving was the swaying. The horizon was moving up and down. The building was designed to swing like a metronome. Japanese engineers believe making a building flexible will keep it upright. There was nothing to do except pray that the engineers knew what they were doing. After about a minute, the horizon stayed still.

We were all stunned and just stared at each other. We turned on the TV and the excited announcer told us that the earthquake was 6 on the Richter scale, the strongest quake in thirteen years. Apart from the elevator being knocked out of service, there was no damage to our building or any other in the neighbourhood. We carried on with our lives, walking down twenty-eight stories. There were fireworks to see.

At one point I wondered if our newscast was somehow connected to a string of oddly timed earthquakes. I concocted the preposterous theory after we had three different earthquakes during three different shows. Each one happened while we were rolling videotape, so the audience was none the wiser. Neither quake was strong enough to send anyone scrambling for cover or even to bother mentioning to the audience, but what a strange coincidence. I mean, three times the earth moved between 8:30 and 8:55 pm Japanese standard time. I asked myself, Does God not like the hosts? Worse, does God not like the English writer from Canada? Whatever the irritant, I just wished that he would stop dropping hints and tell us outright. Perhaps a voice from a burning television. A couple of months later we changed the name of the program. I guess God preferred *News Today: 30 Minutes* to *Newswatch* because we never had another quake during a broadcast.

The most violent earthquake I ever went through was not real. I was in an earthquake simulator operated by the Tokyo Fire Department. I was filming a report on Tokyo's vigilant preparations to be ready for The Big One. The Big One is a monster earthquake, for which Tokyo is long overdue. Japanese scientists predict that it will be apocalyptic in scale. Tens of thousands will die in collapsed buildings and fires.

The earthquake simulator teaches people how to ride out quakes. The accepted wisdom is to stay low, protect your head and get under a table. I actually went through the same thirty-second earthquake twice, for the sake of a television camera. Television likes impressive events shot from different angles. They weren't terrifying because I knew they weren't real, but I was completely helpless. Each time, I started on my knees, holding a pillow over my head. The operator cranked up the tremors to the maximum force. Each time, a foam china cabinet toppled over on me and I fell on my side. The shaking was so savage that my knees and elbows had chafe marks afterwards. It was easy to see how a real quake of that magnitude would kill thousands.

Caring for the survivors is an integral part of Japan's disaster management plan. I was given a tour of a warehouse, just one of many sprinkled around Tokyo, full of supplies to keep survivors of The Big One warm and fed. Thirteen stories of boxes, containing everything from dried food to underwear.

The only thing scarier than being inside a building when The Big One hits is being inside a train hurtling down the tracks. Our crew was invited to film inside the Keikyu Railway Command Center. The centre is connected to seismic equipment that senses shock waves. Depending on the location of a quake's epicentre, the command centre might get just enough of a warning to sound the alarm. A driver would have only seconds to stop his train before the quake knocked it off the tracks.

The Japanese believe in going down fighting, to die with their boots on. Except the Keikyu Railway Command Center doesn't allow outside footwear inside. Everyone has to wear slippers. So if The Big One strikes directly underneath, the dedicated employees of the Keikyu Railway Command Center will die with their slippers on. It doesn't get anymore Japanese than that.

Cancer! What Cancer?

There was something in Dr. Lee's gaze that made me apprehensive. It was early Saturday morning and I had just stepped out of the Georgetown Bakery with an armload of baguettes and croissants. An SUV was coming up the street and Dr. Lee was behind the wheel. St. John's is a small city and I had bumped into Dr. Lee at the bakery once before. He was friendly then. This time he didn't wave. He just briefly stared and drove on.

Dr. Lee's secretary normally had a smile in her voice, but I couldn't detect one during that phone call. This was only a couple of days after the bakery encounter. Dr. Lee wanted to see me.

Dr. Lee had sent my pathology samples to the Armed Forces Institute of Pathology. The AFIP is an agency of the U.S. Department of Defense. When President Abraham Lincoln was assassinated, the forerunner of the AFIP did the autopsy. When the Russian government wanted to confirm the identities of Tsar Nicholas II and the royal family, AFIP scientists assisted. Somewhere in that monstrosity of the AFIP complex in Washington, D.C., was a file with Glenn Deir's name on it. Something didn't add up for Dr. Lee. I had a lump; the St. John's pathology lab couldn't tell him what it was. He wanted an answer.

Deb and I sat outside Dr. Lee's clinic at St. Clare's Hospital. Patient after patient was called in, even those who had registered after me. What was going on? I checked with reception to make sure that my name hadn't slipped through a crack. No, it was there. Dr. Lee wasn't ready for me. After what seemed like an eternity, we were brought in.

Dr. Lee apologized for the delay. "The pathology report has been misplaced. I'm having them fax another, but I didn't want to leave you out there stewing any longer."

He slammed a file shut and slapped it against his thigh. "I'm sorry, but they found a spot of cancer. It's nothing you did or didn't do. It's just shitty luck."

Shitty luck. That's when I knew what a good doctor I had. He was a guy who refused to take no answer as an answer. A guy who cared enough about his patient to send pathology slides to the United States of America for a second opinion. A guy who used gritty English because it suited the occasion. Shitty luck. It should be in medical dictionaries.

I told Dr. Lee, "You were supposed to say, 'You have a benign lump, and it's so special that we're writing it up in a medical journal, calling it Glenn-san Syndrome and you'll never be bothered with it again.'"

"I didn't get the memo," he said with a smile.

"When I told you that you should take your skills and live somewhere else, I was kidding. Don't ... go ... anywhere."

Dr. Lee asked us to wait a while longer while he tracked down the missing pathology report. He left us alone. Deb and I were both stunned and hardly spoke. Cancer. I believed Dr. Lee and yet I didn't. I was as fit as ever. I was running three miles, three mornings a week, and at a good clip. How does a person with cancer do that?

Dr. Lee returned with the fax. He explained that the American pathologists discovered a tiny spot of cancer in one of the three lymph nodes he had taken out of my neck. They were sure of the diagnosis.

"Dr. Lee, what would explain the American pathologists finding cancer and the Newfoundland pathologists missing it?"

"Because," Dr. Lee replied, "they're ..."

Discretion tells me not to reveal what he said because it might cause untold trouble for both of us. Doctors don't like to publicly criticize other doctors. The journalist in me says go on, the patient in me says stop. Patient wins. I like my doctor; I want to keep him.

Dr. Lee was angry because weeks before he had assured me that I was cancer-free, but now he had to take it back. "The Newfoundland medical system is a house of cards," he went on to say.

The American pathologists had even more important news. They were also certain that the cancer in my neck had come from somewhere else. The primary site, the mother ship, was hiding in my body. Dr. Lee would have to hunt for it.

"I'm going to arrange for you to have an MRI," said Dr. Lee.

"Won't that take forever?"

"We'll put in an urgent request. My secretary is good at arranging these things."

"Am I ever glad I was nice to her. I've found that it always pays to be nice to those who sit next to the throne."

"Even if I wanted an MRI for myself I'd have to go through her," said Dr. Lee, powerless against the might of the secretarial Mafia. "I'll also arrange for you to come to the cancer clinic."

Cancer clinic. The words reverberated around my mind. I had walked past its doors a hundred times, never having to contemplate crossing the threshold. Now, those doors were like the River Styx to me. They separated the world of the living from the world of the dead. A grossly unfair portrayal, I realize, but I left Dr. Lee's office thinking, I'll be to hell and back before all this is over.

There was nothing to be gained by being mad at the Newfoundland pathology lab. Really, what had I lost? The delay in treatment could be measured in a few short weeks. It was medically insignificant.

Still, the problems at the lab were supposed to have been

fixed. They had new equipment, new procedures, better training. I had been at a news conference just three months before and heard the chief of laboratory medicine boast that the lab was now as good as any in Canada, if not North America. I even put him in my television report, allowing him to brag to the whole province about achieving a gold standard. If what he said were true, why did they get my diagnosis wrong?

Truth was, my confidence in the pathology lab couldn't fall any lower. It had already been eroded by the harm caused to others. I thought of those breast cancer patients who were in our newscast almost nightly. We were reporting that over an eight-year period a staggering 40 per cent had been given faulty test results. What was negative should have been positive. Those test results were critical in determining the treatment the women received to fight their cancer.

By the time they stopped counting, health officials would discover that over 400 living and dead women had received the wrong diagnosis, and over a hundred of them got the wrong treatment. We'll never know if timely anti-hormonal drugs could have saved the deceased women, but we do know that they never got their chance to fight cancer with the best medicine available.

If anyone had a reason to be full of seething anger, it was those women and their families. At least I would get the right treatment in a reasonable time.

But overriding all those circumstances was a lesson I learned from my sister-in-law, Linda. For three years Linda had reported alarming symptoms to her family doctor, but the doctor didn't pounce on them. Linda continuously felt that her concerns were dismissed. It took a replacement doctor to say, "We'll get to the bottom of this." Eventually, a haematologist diagnosed Linda with stage 4 follicular lymphoma.

Afterwards, Linda went back to her family doctor, wanting to know how she missed the diagnosis. The doctor was devastated by the revelation. What they said to each other has stayed their business, but before Linda left the office she and the doctor hugged. Linda made the noblest decision imaginable: she decided to keep that doctor as her family physician. And with that decision, she discarded the corrosive anger. She opted for reconciliation, not retribution. Linda was able to focus all her energy and strength on the fight ahead. She has never regretted that decision.

Naturally, I wondered how the pathologist in the St. John's lab missed my cancer. Did she have an off day? Did she have the right equipment and training? Did she do all that she should have? I was ticked, but I saw that anger would only gnaw away at me. It was pointless. I decided that, should I ever meet that pathologist, I would simply say, "I just want you to be better at your job."

I might have had cancer, but I still had to eat. Deb brought home sushi-grade tuna. It looked first-rate to me, but I'm no expert. The experts were on the other side of the world in Tokyo's Tsukiji Fish Market.

Tsukiji feeds Tokyo. The warehouses are the size of football fields. People are shouting, front-end loaders are piling up mountains of Styrofoam trays, and carts whiz by at hit & run speed. All before the sun comes up. Live fish, fresh fish, frozen fish, and ugly fish: if it swims in the ocean, you can find it at Tsukiji. And the crown jewel is bluefin tuna.

The tuna are auctioned off to wholesalers every day at 5 am. They are laid out on pallets, hundreds of them. They come from Mexico, the Mediterranean, and God only knows where else. Japan has an insatiable appetite for tuna, so much so that you can have tuna for breakfast just outside the market.

I tagged along with Susumu as he was shooting a story on tuna prices for NHK World. The auction is closed to the public and probably for good reason. There seemed to be at least one buyer for every tuna in the building, so the floor was crowded enough. Non-buyers are simply in the way. I certainly was. I felt something against my leg and looked down to discover that someone had rolled a tuna onto it. I can attest that this is an excellent way to get blood and guts on your jeans. There was no polite, "Sumimasen." *Excuse me.* I got several taps on my back to get out of the way. I was standing between them and profit.

The tools of the trade include a good eye, a flashlight and a hammer-like tool that has a hook instead of a head. The hook is used to open the stomach cavity and the flashlight, of course, gives that good eye a good look. The potential buyer scribbles madly and wanders off to the next batch.

Several auctions happen simultaneously. An auctioneer gathers a crowd by shaking a brass bell. The best auctioneers stand on stools and put on a show. Lots of finger pointing, hand waving, and the Japanese equivalent of, "Who'll give me five, five, five?" They do it with dazzling efficiency. The best tuna that day fetched $10,000. By 6 am, every bluefin is sold and they are being hauled off to market.

Japan eats a quarter of the world's tuna and the Japanese fleet fishes all over the globe. Japan has admitted over-fishing its quota in the past. I'm sure Japan is not alone in its guilt and that every tuna-fishing country is breaking the rules. The stocks are in free-fall. And yet the tuna auction misrepresents the whole crisis. It's vibrant and exciting, and the smell of money is stronger than the smell of fish.

I guess it will be like the northern cod off Newfoundland. One day there won't be anything left to catch.

Cancer killed my mother, it nearly killed my sister Judy, and now it was going to have a crack at me. Telling my sisters about the diagnosis brought back all the fear and anxiety we had lived through years before. My own family had already shown me that cancer is a fickle disease. It capriciously decided to let Judy live, and Mom die. Flip a coin. Heads Glenn lives, tails Glenn dies. Is that what it would come down to?

Deb and I walked to the cancer clinic. I had a sense it would

SICK JOKE

be a day of destiny; this was the day I would hear the good, the bad and the ugly. After registering at the front desk, we were directed to chairs off to the side. I glanced up from a magazine and spied Dr. Lee bolting for the front door. I wanted to call out, "Where the hell are you going?" but he was focused on his pager. There was obviously some emergency and I wouldn't be seeing him.

Our next stop was downstairs. Could the architect not have foreseen the obvious symbolism of descending into the inferno? The damned sat on deceivingly comfortable chairs waiting for Lucifer's agents, disguised as sweet nurses, to call them into the fiery pit. The devil didn't wear Prada. She wore a stethoscope.

That's the Evil Glenn talking. To be fair, the cancer clinic contains radiation bunkers, with bunkers being the operative word. They use high-density concrete in the walls and ceiling to contain the radiation. You can't easily put that weight on the upper floors. It would be wrong of me to argue that nothing good ever happened in a bunker. Adolf Hitler committed suicide in his.

Deb and I fretted in an examination room. There was a knock on the door and in marched the medical SWAT team. Four people at once. That's when the seriousness of my predicament hit me. There was a round of handshakes and introductions. Dr. Ken Burrage was a head and neck surgeon; Dr. Alia Norman a radiation oncologist. The entourage included an oncology nurse and a medical student.

Dr. Burrage went first. Whenever a doctor puts on latex gloves you just know that it's not going to be comfortable. Fortunately, he wasn't a proctologist.

"Open wide," said Dr. Burrage, as he jammed his index finger as far as he could into the back of my throat and felt around. I gagged, sneezed, and coughed. This search for my primary cancer was a little less high-tech than I had imagined. It was a good old-fashioned physical exam; the complete opposite of an MRI scan.

Dr. Lee's secretary had indeed worked her magic and found an MRI slot for me. It was like lying down inside a video game. The whirl, pings, pops and bangs were deafening. No wonder they gave me earplugs. The MRI produced stunningly clear, 3-D images of the inside of my head and neck, but no sign of anything that didn't belong.

I was headed back to the operating room. Dr. Burrage said they needed to put a scope deep into my throat, voice box and lungs to have a look around. Plus they wanted biopsies. They intended to snip a piece from the base of my tongue, another from a cavity in my throat, a third from behind my nose, and then take out my left tonsil. Not both tonsils, just the left. The one closest to the spot in my neck where the original lump had been.

"Let me see if I've got this right," I said. "I'm forty-nine years old and you're going to take out my tonsil."

"Ya," said Dr. Burrage.

"Do I get all the ice cream I want?"

Dr. Burrage smirked. It was the sly smile that has disguised the lie doctors have been telling tonsillectomy patients forever. "Oh ya." He nodded and the smirk widened.

"We'll do this Friday," said Dr. Burrage. This was Tuesday, only three days warning.

"Is there any chance this can be moved? We have a family function on Friday." Deb and I had planned to join her clan for a BBQ at the cottage.

"No, I have to move people around to get you in."

The battle was lost. Friday it would be. Dr. Burrage excused himself and Dr. Norman stepped forward. She began by explaining that surgery alone probably wouldn't keep the cancer at bay. I would need radiation treatment on my head or neck no matter what they found on Friday. Even if they didn't find anything, radiation was the recommended treatment.

There would be an avalanche of side effects. I would lose my taste, my saliva would turn rope-like and then disappear altogether, my beard wouldn't grow, my skin would turn sunburn red, my throat was going to get so sore that I'd be able to eat only soft food, and I'd be at high risk for tooth decay.

"We can protect your teeth. See your dentist and get her to

make fluoride trays." Whatever the hell fluoride trays were I was going to be getting them.

"Will my taste ever come back?"

"Yes, but it's never quite the same." Her lip trembled a little. I wondered if I was making her nervous.

"What about the sunburn?"

"It will fade in time. Your skin will look normal, but you'll probably have a little of this." Dr. Norman pinched her neck and jiggled it. "It shouldn't be too noticeable, but I can always tell when someone has had radiation. Your beard will come back, but it will probably be blotchy."

How could people who spoke so gently want to hurt me so much? Weren't these the same people who took an oath of "Do No Harm?" My treatment would prove the cliché that the cure is worse than the disease.

"What are the odds of getting rid of the cancer permanently?"

"There's a 90 per cent chance of a cure. There's a 10 per cent chance it could come back. Higher than the average person on the street who has never had cancer, but good odds."

"And if I don't have radiation?"

"There's a 40 per cent chance the cancer will return."

Choice, what choice? It sounded to me that if I refused the radiation I might as well sign my own death warrant.

Deb was sobbing. I held her hand as she dabbed her eyes with a tissue. I felt terrible. A husband is supposed to protect his wife, not make her cry. I couldn't stop what these doctors had started. I was powerless. How many times had the doctors and nurses seen this drama? The devastated couple — bewildered, overwhelmed, brittle.

I was particularly worried about my voice. You can't be a television reporter if your voice is raspy or your mouth is so dry that you can't form words properly.

"Would you be willing to travel?" asked Dr. Norman. "Princess Margaret Hospital in Toronto has specialized radiation. They might be able to save your salivary glands."

There was a glimmer of hope that I wouldn't be cursed with dry mouth for the rest of my days.

"I can afford it."

"I have to talk to my boss and if he approves, we'll see if Toronto will take you. They usually do when we ask."

We were left alone. I put my arm around Deb. We didn't speak. It was my darkest day as a cancer patient. They were indeed going to fling me into the fiery pit. They promised to get me out again, but it would be a painful climb.

It was time to leave. "Good thing I brought sunglasses," said Deb as she covered her bloodshot eyes.

We walked out of the cancer clinic into a gorgeous, blue-sky day. We decided to drive to St. Philip's for a meal of fish and chips. Shag healthy food. Fat lot of good that had done me. Cholesterol was no longer the worry it had been. Alas, the restaurant saved me from myself. It was closed. We settled for turkey sandwiches from the corner store.

We sat on a large beach rock overlooking Conception Bay. The water lapped at the shoreline. We reconstructed the morning's events and conversations. So much information, so fast. There were gaps, questions not asked.

An oil rig was anchored off Bell Island. It was the symbol of so much promise for my home province. Oil prices were skyrocketing. Newfoundland and Labrador was collecting barrels of money in royalties. Premier Brian Peckford's prediction twenty-five years earlier — "One day the sun will shine and have-not will be no more" — was on the verge of coming true. Despite the optimistic prognosis, I had misgivings about whether I would be around to see it happen.

I vowed that day never to ask the question, "Why me?" The right question was, "Why the hell not me?" Better men than I have had their lives taken prematurely.

Scott was my best friend in high school and university. He

died from a blood clot in a lung, the last domino to fall in a series that began with a ruptured brain aneurysm. I delivered the eulogy at his funeral in front of his widow, three sons and a packed church in our hometown of Grand Falls-Windsor.

Bryan was my best friend when we lived in Halifax. He died from cancer. It began as melanoma — skin cancer — that spread throughout his body. I mourned him by contemplating our friendship at a Buddhist shrine in Tokyo.

Bryan and Scott never met each other, but each had a laugh that brightened my life immeasurably. They were good men, outstanding men, and if Fate or God could take them before their time, then I was not entitled to any self-pity.

I had a phone call to make. I dialled my boss's number.

"Janice, I won't be back to work today. In fact I won't be back to work for a couple of weeks at least."

"Glenn, are you all right?"

"No, Janice, I'm not. I'm not all right. In the short term, I may get back to work for a while and then I'll be gone again. In the long term, you'd better find someone else to cover the Liberals during the election. I won't be able to do it."

The provincial election was only six weeks away on October 9. Janice had offered me the chance to ride the Liberal campaign bus. Election travel is a perk and one of the best for a local television reporter. I was so looking forward to it. Three weeks of visiting the most beautiful nooks and crannies in Newfoundland and Labrador, and CBC's dime would pay for it. The Liberals were manning the barricades, desperately trying to ward off annihilation by Premier Danny Williams and his Conservative government. Now someone else would have to chronicle the Liberals' last stand. Cancer was already stealing things from me.

"Take care of yourself, Glenn, get better." Janice laughed nervously. Perhaps I sounded like I was at death's door and she was terribly uncomfortable. She wouldn't be the last person to feel nervous and uncomfortable around me.

Sometimes the darkest hours can produce the blackest humour. After our afternoon on the beach, Deb went to visit her parents. During my two years in Japan, Deb's father had stored my hunting rifle. He had been meaning to return it for some time, but kept forgetting. Just before Deb was about to leave, Jim's memory synapses sparked.

Give Glenn back his gun, he thought.

Jim was far from unkind. He was as concerned about my health as anyone in the family. But *Return Glenn's Gun* was on his to-do list and here was an easy way to accomplish that. In Old School Newfoundland, guns are not about murder or self-destruction. They are about hunting, and they are prized possessions. Carrying my gun case, Deb waved goodbye to her parents.

Return Glenn's Gun. Done.

By the time she walked through our front door, Deb, normally very much her father's daughter on such pragmatic matters, was struck by the raw irony of giving a man his rifle on the day he gets the grimmest news of his life. She dropped the gun case in the front hall and cried out, "If you do anything to hurt yourself with this gun, I'll never forgive myself."

I could do nothing but laugh at the absurdity of it all. Of course, there was always an outside chance that the Youden clan was indeed suggesting that I shouldn't be a burden on the family. That this whole cancer thing was going to be too much of a bother for everyone and therefore I should go off to the woods, "make away with myself," as they say in Old School Newfoundland, and don't leave a mess for anyone else to clean up. Possibly, but not likely. Jim Youden is an avid outdoorsman. Maybe, just maybe, Jim's real view was that nothing cheers up a depressed hunter like a reunion with his Thirty-Aught-Six.

My Left Tonsil

Question 29 stopped me dead in my tracks. I was in St. Clare's Hospital for a pre-operation clinic. The idea was to make sure that I wouldn't die on the table while they were taking out my tonsil. Of course they wanted my medical history. I was given a long questionnaire to complete. Heart trouble, mental illness, seizures? No, no, no. Every answer was no. I was breezing through. I was checking the no boxes with flair. But my cockiness ended with question 29. Do you have, or have you had, cancer? Yes. It was the first time in my life that I had to answer yes to that question.

I got a quick physical from the doctor. "You're a healthy man," he said.

"Healthy as a horse — except I have cancer."

I could say the words without tripping over them, but they didn't belong in *my* mouth, did they? Sadly, they did. I would have to get used to saying them.

Of all places to run into someone I knew — the day surgery prep room. What are the odds? I used to work with her at CBC years before. We were friendly to each other, but not friends. It had been a while since I had seen her. But there we were, both in johnny coats, waiting to be wheeled into operating rooms. I decided to employ elevator etiquette. Extend common courtesies, yes, but not engage in conversation. I nodded hello to my old CBC colleague, and avoided shouting out, "I'm here to see if they can find my cancer. What about you?"

Everyone says getting your tonsils out is more painful as an adult. I guess I should have had the right tonsil out as a kid and then I would have been in the perfect position to compare. The hospital's tonsillectomy brochure was silent on the debate. It did promise me pain though, and it advised me to take my medication every four hours.

Just as before, Deb walked me to the doors of the operating room. We were both calm. This would be a search mission only, and would not evolve into a search and destroy mission. I would leave the operating room with the same neck and facial features that I entered with.

The anaesthetist warmed up the crowd by saying, "I can't make out the writing. Your age, is that forty-nine or ninety-nine?" He gave me a nudge on the arm. I thought, Oh great, Henny Youngman is going to knock me out.

A nurse snorted when she saw the dust and pollen allergy warning on my chart. "Yet another man who has found a way to get out of housework. It's a scam, isn't it?"

I wondered whether someone had stuck a "Kick me" sign on my back. Another nurse asked what I did for a living. "This is distressing," I said. "I'm a reporter, I'm frequently on TV and this tells me that you're watching the other God-damn guys."

Oh no, they all protested. No time to watch television news of any sort. I guess they're too busy mocking the patients. I got no relief until I was comatose.

I awoke with a burning sensation in the back of my throat and the nurse gave me some liquid painkiller. I was groggy when Dr. Burrage stopped by. His news was really no news. There was nothing obvious in my esophagus, larynx or lungs. They looked perfectly normal. The cancer was doing a fine job of hiding. He hoped to have the pathology reports on the biopsies for the following Tuesday, when I would go to the cancer clinic again.

They kept me in the recovery room for four hours, just long enough to make sure that I wouldn't haemorrhage to death. By late afternoon I was sitting in an Adirondack chair in my backyard sipping a cold drink. Life was still good.

The doctor ordered a liquid and soft food diet for two weeks. I could try flaky fish after five days, but definitely no chicken, beef or pork until fourteen days after the operation. They needn't have worried about me defying their directions. I was in good shape, but whenever I swallowed, it felt like someone was rubbing the back of my throat with sandpaper. I couldn't imagine swallowing if both tonsils had been removed.

The culinary torture actually started as I was coming out of the anaesthetic. I was dreaming about carving a roast coated in Szechwan peppercorns. The reality couldn't have been more different. That night's supper consisted of beef broth. It was served in a two-handle china bowl, but it was still measly beef broth. The next morning I had Cream of Wheat. Deb also had a serving out of sympathy.

"I had forgotten how much I like this," she said.

"I had forgotten how much I hate this," I replied. It was going to be a *long* fourteen days.

I found myself thinking of another former premier: Joey Smallwood. My earliest memory of Joey was actually of a Joey impersonator. I was a child, perhaps no more than seven, attending a play in the basement of the Grand Falls United Church. An actor wearing horn-rimmed glasses strolled onto the stage and someone yelled, "It's Joey." A titter rippled through the audience. The boss of the province, the man my parents faithfully voted for, was there and everyone had better be on his or her best behaviour. Despite my tender years, I knew Joey Smallwood was someone to be feared and revered.

I met the real Joey Smallwood early in my journalism career. He was no longer the premier, but he still commanded a role in Newfoundland politics, albeit from the sidelines. Joey had been subpoenaed to testify into an investigation of fraud and stock manipulation, dating back to his days as premier. Joey was fighting the subpoena, claiming cabinet secrecy.

It was a wholly impenetrable story for television. The events were more than a decade old, they happened behind closed doors and were never filmed, Joey himself was not accused of wrongdoing, and stock manipulations are notoriously complicated at the best of times. Still, Joey's stature made the story impossible to ignore. My assignment was to interview the former premier and deliver a two-minute-ish story.

Joey proceeded to give me a lecture on constitutional law and how cabinet ministers enjoyed blanket immunity from prying eyes. My eyes were glazing over. Joey was filling my videotape with numbing details. I needed a "We'll fight them on the beaches" clip. Emotion is the lifeblood of television. Without it, my story would be terminally boring.

"Mr. Smallwood, can we just jump to the message you want to send to those investigators?"

Joey scowled at me. "Don't push me, boy. All my life *I've* done the pushing and you're not going to push me around." It was definitely "boy" that he said. Not "b'y," that informal term of address that I had taught Susumu in Tokyo. This "boy" had a condescending tone. A superior was talking to a subordinate, a person with a lower station in life.

I immediately imagined my career in flames. Joey was a good friend of the television station owner. Back then I worked for NTV — a private company. It lacked the journalistic fortress that CBC, a Crown corporation, gives its reporters. NTV would kowtow to irritated advertisers by killing or ignoring embarrassing stories. Politicians saw NTV as a transcription service. Our tiny newsroom had neither the experience nor the gumption to pry deeply into political affairs. All Joey had to do was make a well-placed phone call and I'd be unceremoniously marched into the station manager's office. Joey ran Newfoundland virtually unchallenged for twenty-two years. On that day, Joey behaved like the autocratic premier and I had better do what I was told. I dutifully listened, at great length, to what he had to say and politely thanked him for his time before scurrying away like a kicked dog.

I met Joey Smallwood one more time before he died. It was 1987. By then he had suffered a debilitating stroke. This charismatic orator, this man who could hold an audience spellbound, this man who convinced a people to forsake their own country and join another, could barely speak.

Joey was a thrilling speaker during the Confederation debate. Whenever I heard the old radio broadcasts I admired his mastery of English. It was beautifully simple, designed to evoke emotions and persuade. He delivered the words with clarity and bravado. Joey's passion may have been contrived, nothing more than political opportunism, but could he ever hold your attention. His 1946 speech pleading with Newfoundlanders to rally around Confederation was brilliant.

> *Compared with the mainland of North America, we are 50 years, in some things 100 years, behind the times. We live more poorly, more shabbily, more meanly. Our life is more a struggle. Our struggle is tougher, more naked, more hopeless ... We all love this land. It has charm that warms our hearts, go where we will; a charm, a magic, a mystical tug on our emotion that never dies. With all her faults, we love her.* (Canadian Parliamentary Review, V. 15(2), 1992)

Forty-one years later, the great debater and braggart was almost silent. Joey was attending an event to receive donations to a trust fund bearing his name. The fund was set up to help Smallwood finish his great passion after retiring from politics: *The Encyclopedia of Newfoundland and Labrador.* An Ontario man named Bill Mole was presenting him with cheques totalling around $1500. Mole had walked across Newfoundland gathering donations along the way.

Joey had fallen on hard times. Two months earlier, a sheriff had served him with a court order demanding that he pay unpaid publishing bills. The spectacle was caught by CBC's cameras and broadcast across the country. The video of this broken man spawned fundraisers of every shape and description.

Joey was mute during the cheque presentation, but he agreed to a radio interview with me afterwards. He was gaunt, a pitiful sight. I crafted my questions to allow for yes or no answers. I asked if the donations would encourage others to give? He surprised me by speaking the words "Hope so." He struggled to get that simple phrase out. Fate had capriciously taken away the thing he loved the most — talking.

As I contemplated my cancer diagnosis, it occurred to me that Joey Smallwood and I shared the same whims of destiny. Fate was going to cruelly take something away from me too, one of my greatest pleasures, the taste of food. The delights of the palate were a serious pursuit to me. Whether it was lemon chicken in Hanoi, barbequed beef in Seoul, Peking duck in Beijing or caribou stew in St. John's, my taste buds were well treated around the world. Hot, sour, salt and sweet were all welcome in my mouth. And I was on the verge of losing the ability to enjoy them all.

Radiation damages taste buds. During the full weight of the radiation onslaught, food might taste like cardboard or nothing at all. The medical literature told me that some people recover their taste a few months after therapy ends. But for many, the change is permanent. Blueberries might never taste like blueberries again.

While medical gore has never unsettled my stomach, I could never be a doctor. Everyone who comes into your office has a problem. I'm not that understanding or compassionate. I could be a nurse though; in fact I was one in Japan.

One Sunday I linked up with Michael, a Brit who came to Japan for just a couple of years about twenty-five years earlier. Michael was a hiker extraordinaire. He had walked thousands of miles over hill and dale in Japan, and published two hiking books. I figured I was in good hands.

We caught the first morning bullet train out of Tokyo bound for Nagano, host of the 1998 Winter Olympics. From there it was onto a local train and then a bus up into the mountains. Our final destination was Mount Kurohime. The goal was not to reach the peak, rather we intended to walk a trail around it, about three-quarters of the way up.

We spent the first two hours climbing. There was quite a bit of huffing and puffing. It's a good thing Michael has a pacemaker or I wouldn't have been able to keep up. Every so often, when he overexerted himself, his pacemaker would drop his heart rate. He'd have to take a breather and naturally, so did I. You see, I couldn't abandon my patient. I was his "nurse." Well, that's what we told Japan Rail anyway. It got me a discount ticket. As a "disabled" person Michael is entitled to cheaper fares and the benefit extends to his medical assistant. Hence, I was Nurse Deir.

Michael speaks and reads Japanese fluently. "What does that sign say?" I asked.

"Be careful. You're in bear country." Who knew? Japan has a black bear population. Michael attached a bell to his knapsack to alert the bears to our presence. Hopefully, they would scurry away and not announce, "Dinner's coming." Michael and I kidded each other about whom the bear would get first.

"I don't have to outrun the bear," I said. "I only have to outrun you. And with your pacemaker, that shouldn't be too much of a problem."

I guess I'm more Nurse Ratched than Nurse Deir.

●

Why do women treat the men in their lives with complete contempt? I mean, how does a woman go from hanging onto her man's every word, to not listening to a single word he says? Worse still, if the words are heard, they are held up to ridicule and scorn. The venue matters not. Case in point — the Dr. H. Bliss Murphy Cancer Centre.

I had come again hoping to discover where my primary cancer was hiding. Deb was with me and so was her sister Karen. We asked Karen to come along to act as a note-taker. Deb and I realized during our first visit to the clinic that information was coming at us so furiously that we couldn't take it all in.

We were waiting for the doctors in an examination room, discussing the Internet research I had done on the radiation treatment offered at Princess Margaret Hospital in Toronto. It's called Intensity-Modulated Radiation Therapy, commonly shortened to IMRT. IMRT is a type of 3-D radiation treatment that delivers different doses of x-rays to small areas of tissue from different angles. A tumour receives higher doses, while nearby healthy tissue receives lower doses or none at all. Older radiation techniques and machines tend to take the shotgun approach, sending out a wide blast. Cancerous cells and healthy cells get the same full-strength dosage. IMRT is more rifle-like. A single shot to a specific target. IMRT hits the bull's-eye with thin beams of radiation. It usually produces fewer side effects.

There was a chance that Princess Margaret could save the glands that produce saliva, protect my voice box, and burn less of my neck and face. All vital anatomical parts in my line of work. I was acutely aware of the whimsical critiques of television audiences. Female journalists suffer from far more catty chatter about their appearance than male journalists, but men on camera ignore personal appearance at their peril. Your clothes, hair, face and voice must not be distracting; otherwise people won't hear a single word you're saying. Vanity, thy name is TV reporter.

So much to ponder; so much to worry about. You'd think

that a guy in my circumstances could have counted on the women closest to him for unflinching support. But oooohhhh nooooo! That was asking for too much.

"I hope the Toronto option comes through," I said. "I make my living with my voice and my looks."

Deb and Karen glanced at each other and burst into gales of laughter. Great guffaws. Cackles. The two of them. They were in full howl when the doctors marched in. No man is a god to his wife, or to his sister-in-law apparently.

Dr. Boyd Lee was back with the medical team. I was glad even though I had no qualms about Dr. Ken Burrage. I felt I had a better rapport with Dr. Lee. Maybe it was because I started with him, or maybe it was because he laughed at my jokes. I kidded him about being tossed between doctors like a hot potato. "You take him. No no, you take him." He assured me that wasn't the situation.

Unfortunately, the pathology reports weren't ready but would be soon. It was deflating. I was promised a phone call later in the afternoon. The group was as anxious as I was to get the results of the biopsies and tonsillectomy. The mother cancer is found 98 per cent of the time, and since everything else came up negative, the laboratory would likely solve the mystery.

While that nugget of information would have to wait, the check-up was wonderfully illuminating in another way. The look of surprise on Dr. Lee's face when he heard that only my left tonsil had been removed told me that he would have done things very differently in the operating room.

"You would have taken both tonsils?"

Dr. Lee nodded yes. Clearly he was a guy who liked to cut away any potential danger. But just as clearly, Dr. Burrage didn't see any danger in leaving the right tonsil behind. I had just witnessed medicine cross from science into art, a glimpse of the medical head-butting that usually happens behind closed doors.

I asked, "Are we okay with this?"

Dr. Lee glanced at Dr. Alia Norman, the radiation oncologist. She quickly said that she didn't see the need for any more surgery. She was convinced that radiation would stop the cancer dead in its tracks. Dr. Lee didn't argue. It was medicine by committee, a united position in front of the patient.

I thought of Bob Wakeham, a former colleague at CBC television. He had battled cancer a couple of times, the last battle requiring the wisdom of Solomon to resolve. On one hand, Bob had a radiologist telling him that cancer had returned to his liver and he would soon die. On the other hand, he had a surgeon telling him that the shadows on his scans were nothing more than scar tissue. It took exploratory surgery to end the debate, and thankfully the surgeon was right.

No doubt, it's sometimes difficult to get unanimity between specialists. I had to remind myself that they were giving me their best guess — an educated guess, but a guess nonetheless.

We spent a lot of time reviewing what I could expect in Toronto and the merits of IMRT. The St. John's cancer clinic did a little IMRT but it was reserved for special cases, such as a tumour around an eye. St. John's had neither the personnel nor equipment to offer universal IMRT.

I still held out a faint hope that radiation could be avoided. It was a foolish notion really. "Are you sure I should have radiation?"

"Glenn, if the cancer comes back in your neck, it won't be pretty," said Dr. Lee. "It definitely won't be pretty."

Dr. Norman reminded me that without radiation there was a 40 per cent chance that the cancer would return. It was possible that cancer cells had already established another nest in my neck. No eye could see it, no test could detect it. By having radiation there was a 90 per cent chance that I would be cured. Cured! I liked the sound of that. I mentally waved the white flag. There was nothing to do except wait for Toronto to call. I would have to drop everything at a moment's notice and go.

It was a fitful afternoon. I paced around the house waiting for Dr. Norman to call with the pathology report. Then I had a pleasant surprise from friends in London, England. An arrangement of flowers was delivered to my door. There were roses, sunflowers and some purple flowers that resembled fire pokers.

After two hours of nothing, the phone rang the same instant as the doorbell rang. I had Dr. Norman on the phone and the flower delivery guy at the door, again. Yet *another* bouquet from my friends in London. I was flabbergasted. Two! When I got back to the phone I joked with Dr. Norman about all the flowers. "I'm not dead yet." I found out later that it was a mistake. Cathy and Ned like me, but not two arrangements' worth.

"Mr. Deir, they found cancer in your tonsil," said Dr. Norman. "All the other biopsies came back negative."

Tonsil cancer! I had never heard of such a thing. Dr. Norman had of course. It was uncommon, but when you're in Dr. Norman's line of work you see it from time to time.

My left tonsil was the primary source of the cancer that showed up in my neck. I had something called "a poorly differentiated carcinoma." And my cancer was being classified as "T1N2b." Dr. Norman explained what that meant, but it was like she was speaking a different language. I'd have to look it up later on the Internet and absorb the information a little bit at a time.

I asked Dr. Norman if she had confidence in the pathology. Were they sure? She said yes.

Dr. Norman said I had every reason to be optimistic. They had caught the cancer early and it was only on the surface of the tonsil. What a relief that it hadn't bored deep inside. My margins, the tissue closest to other parts of my throat, were clean. The cancer consisted of islands and nests of cells in the tonsil. Apparently, they had made part of the tonsil surface go hard. Impossible for a doctor to see when he's peering into a mouth with the naked eye because the tonsil has an irregular surface anyway, and it's partially hidden back there. The doctor only gets a good look when he cuts it out and puts a piece under a microscope.

A poorly differentiated carcinoma. What a loser. I couldn't even get something that easily rolled off my cancer-free tongue.

Alien Invasion

"Who the hell gets tonsil cancer?" wrote my cousin Ann from faraway Hamilton, Ontario. "This just confirms to me that you will do anything to get attention!"

Ann and I had been friends since we were kids. She had my blessing to make fun of me any time she wanted. Plus, she knew firsthand what was coming my way. Ann had lost both of her breasts because of cancer. The flippant remark was her reminder to hang onto my sense of humour. I was going to need it.

When friends bump into you on the street and ask, "What's new?" they don't really expect you to reply, "Well I just found out that I've got cancer." And yet that's what they got from me in the days immediately after my diagnosis. There seemed to be no easy way to soften the news. As soon as I mentioned the dreaded "C" word, jaws would drop.

People were naturally flummoxed and shocked. There were countless "I am so sorry," "I don't know what to say," and disbelieving exclamations of "Tonsil cancer!" All of which was perfectly understandable. I answered questions as plainly as I could, but tried not to drown my friends in information. I let them set the pace. Some people had a dozen questions, others only one or two. I found telling them that I was going to be okay after treatment took the tension out of the air.

Inevitably, these awkward sidewalk chats drifted into a story about Uncle So-and-So who survived prostate or some other cancer about as anatomically unconnected to one's tonsil as you could imagine. I never took offence. People were nervously volunteering their idea of a pep talk. They meant to offer me hope. I tended to see the black humour in it. I fantasized that they were suggesting that irradiating my posterior would be good for tonsil cancer.

I did get some odd reactions though, again out of nervousness. One friend offered to give me her chiropractor's name. "Saved me from seven whiplashes," she said. I was so stunned I forgot to ask what in heaven's name she was doing to have nearly seven whiplashes. I couldn't help myself; I laughed. She later wrote a note apologizing. She really didn't need to. No offence was taken.

Another friend hit me with some biting humour about having a lecherous desire to hang around nurses, and suggested I should apply for a job in Washington with Al Jazeera. Can a new job cure cancer? My witty email had obviously done too good a job of masking the seriousness of my situation.

My sister Barb went speechless during our phone conversation. I could hear her draw on a cigarette. "Phyllis down the road had two brain tumours removed this year." She had another puff. "They say that she's all right, but I don't believe it." Thank God I wasn't Phyllis.

I had two phone calls that lifted my spirits. Peter and Con knew firsthand what lay ahead. Both had been through neck surgery and radiation treatment. Peter had tongue cancer and Con had a cancerous lump in his neck. At least their cancers were in the ballpark, so I paid close attention.

Neither man tried to sugarcoat the side effects. Con said if the doctors ever wanted to irradiate his neck again he wouldn't let them. I found out much later that irradiating the mouth and neck twice is not medically possible, but I got Con's point. He'd sooner die than go through it again.

Con had a warning for me about the radiation. "For the first two weeks, I had no side effects. I was thinking, If that's the worst you can do to me, bring it on." He grew to regret his cockiness. Towards the end of his treatment he would feel sick just driving to the hospital.

"Glenn, think of me as the canary in the coal mine," said Con. "If I dropped dead right now, you'd still have nine years." That's how long Con had been cancer-free.

To celebrate being cancer-free for two years, Peter and two friends (Deb's brother being one) cross-country skied sixty kilometres through the wilderness of Newfoundland's Avalon Peninsula. Over four days they had whiteout conditions, freezing rain, bitter winds, a little sunshine and the time of their lives.

"I'm more active now than before I had cancer," Peter told me.

They wanted to perk me up and they did. They were living proof that good days would follow bad.

For a man whose first language is Japanese, Okawa-san has a wonderful way with English. He can turn a phrase. He was unintentionally funny when he first heard about my medical trouble. He advised me, "Please take care of yourself and do not quarrel with Debbie-san. Family peace comes first for recuperation." Apparently, Debbie-san could quarrel with me all she wanted, but Glenn-san had to bite his tongue. I wonder what the Japanese is for "Yes, dear. Whatever you say, dear."

After the cancer diagnosis had been confirmed and the decision made that I would need a tonsillectomy, Okawa-san wrote, "We are really sorry that you have to receive an operation and be treated by radiation to fight against aliens in your body." An English speaker couldn't have said it any better. Cancer was an alien in my body.

The word alien has a specific meaning in Japan. It means a foreigner who is legally allowed to live in Japan. I was an "alien" in Tokyo. By law I had to carry a Certificate of Alien Registration at all times and show it to the police whenever they demanded, though they never bothered me. I liked Okawa-san's concept. Did the cancer cells have a Certificate of Alien Registration and a multiple re-entry permit from the immigration bureau in Shinagawa district? I'd show them mine if they'd show me theirs. When Toronto was done with me, the Certificate of Alien Registration and re-entry permit should be permanently revoked.

I was peeling a mango when Dr. Lee's words took on frightening clarity. "Glenn, if the cancer comes back in your neck, it won't be pretty. It definitely won't be pretty."

The mango was a little soft. I could make indentations when I squeezed it. The peel was unblemished; it was green with a splash of red. All the signs pointed to a succulent mango.

I cut the peel and discovered that the surface fruit was overripe and spoiled. I thought, No problem, I'll just cut away the mottled mango and find edible yellow mango beneath. I sliced and sliced and sliced. I tried the other side of the mango. I cut until all I had left was the pit. There was no healthy mango, just diseased mango.

I realized if the cancer came back in my neck, Dr. Lee could only cut away a small part and then he'd have to stop. Unlike my surgery on the mango, he couldn't keep cutting until there was nothing left. He'd have to close me up and advise me to get my affairs in order. No, it wouldn't be pretty at all.

Toronto would see a much slimmer Glenn Deir. Eating food from a blender and no alcohol had trimmed ten pounds from my physique. It occurred to me that there was a fortune to be made here. If I could package Dr. Deir's Tonsillectomy Diet, I'd be rich. Guaranteed to lose ten pounds in a week or your money back. And just as your throat is healing you can have the second tonsil removed and lose another ten pounds. Overweight people would be beating a path to my door.

Forget the Atkins and Scarsdale diets. I had discovered the next great fad diet. I'd be famous and rich. Oprah would have me on her show, probably next to Tom Cruise jumping on the couch. This cancer thing could pay dividends.

I spent hours on the Internet trying to figure out how exactly I got tonsil cancer. But finding anything specific on tonsil cancer was a challenge all by itself. There is plenty to read about head and neck cancers, but that's where the real detective work starts.

Tonsil cancer is usually lumped in with oropharyngeal cancer, that's cancer found at the back of the mouth. It includes the soft roof of the mouth, the back third of the tongue, the side and back walls of the throat, and the tonsils. This might make perfect sense to doctors, but it was maddening to me. While I was sympathetic to people with palate and tongue cancers, I wanted a library dedicated to my cancer alone and it just wasn't there.

Still, I was able to glean a few facts about tonsil cancer. According to the National Cancer Institute in the United States, if you take 100,000 people, one and a half of them will get tonsil cancer in any given year. (I guess I was the half because I had cancer in only one tonsil.) And every year tonsil cancer will kill one person out of seven diagnosed with it.

Most of the time I had to be satisfied with information about oropharyngeal cancer. I thought it's appropriately named because it's certainly a mouthful to say. Or-oh-fuh-rin-jee-ul. I mastered the pronunciation, but to what end? I might impress a doctor, but friends would surely be baffled. Tonsil cancer was much easier to understand.

I discovered that men get oropharyngeal cancer five times more frequently than women. And it typically strikes between ages fifty and eighty. I was forty-nine. On those points I matched the profile of the textbook patient. But on many others I couldn't have been more different.

I don't smoke. I'm not a heavy drinker. (Full disclosure demands that I admit to the odd binge weekend, like the time friends and I taste-tested our way through the entire inventory of sake in a Tokyo restaurant and then finished the carousing with beer at a pub.) I eat lots of fruits and vegetables daily. I don't drink a South American concoction called mate, and I don't chew that Asian favourite of fresh areca nuts wrapped in betel leaves.

But I do like sex. The literature talked of a link between oropharyngeal cancer and the human papillomavirus. HPV is often passed from one person to another by sexual contact, and is better known for causing cervical cancer. I didn't know if I was HPV positive or not, but it seemed the most likely suspect. Nothing else made sense.

The more sex partners a person has, the more likely he or she can pick up HPV. I wryly said to Deb, "I know *I've* been faithful. Is there something you'd like to confess now?" She gave me a withering look.

If HPV were the culprit, Dr. Lee would be absolutely right. My getting tonsil cancer was "shitty luck" indeed.

T1N2b. It was time to unravel that bit of medical jargon.

I faintly hoped that T1N2b was a Borg designation. I imagined myself sliding up to Seven of Nine in a bar saying, "I'm T1N2b. Assimilate here often?" Alas, it was all in vain. Medical literature can be so boring.

T1N2b simply referred to the severity or extent of my cancer. T stands for tumour. T1 meant that when they measured the tumour in my tonsil the biggest part was 2 cm across, or less. Mine was actually 1 cm. N stands for node, as in lymph node. N2b meant that the cancer had travelled to multiple lymph nodes on one side of my neck. That struck me as wrong because the pathologist had found only one spot of cancer in one lymph node. Eventually, my cancer was labelled T1N1, with N1 meaning the cancer travelled to just a single lymph node. Dr. Deir was right.

Put it all together and it meant that I was either a bad stage 2 or a good stage 3 cancer patient, depending on your perspective. Stage 1 is the best; stage 4 is the worst. I was floating around the middle of the pack.

A poorly differentiated carcinoma. That was the other medical jargon that Dr. Norman had dropped into my hands. Carcinoma I knew. It was a fancy word for cancer. Poorly differentiated I had to look up. A dictionary of cancer terms said poorly differentiated cells lack the structure of normal cells and grow uncontrollably. They reminded me of Borg nanoprobes. I might be able to work that into a Seven of Nine pickup line.

I have been to the mountaintop. Often that phrase is a metaphor for some epiphany, but in my case it's a literal statement. I climbed to the top of Mt. Fuji, Fuji-san to the Japanese — the most celebrated, revered, photographed, painted and highest mountain in all of Japan. Its symmetrical cone shape stands 3776 metres tall and is snow-capped for all but three months of the year. Fuji-san is a glorious sight, no matter what the season. I had made the climb exactly one year before in September 2006. The first anniversary of any event seems to evoke reflection and I was wallowing in it. It was far more pleasurable than sorting through the intricacies of cancer.

To be completely honest, climbing Mt. Fuji is not like climbing Mt. Everest. Mt. Fuji is less than half the height, and one does not need oxygen, ropes, ice picks or Sherpa guides. It's more of a hike than a climb, but climb sounds so much more impressive and gives one delusions about being a mountaineer; 200,000 people "climb" Fuji-san every year, everyone from grandkids to grandparents. So my accomplishment was not heroic in the Sir Edmund Hillary tradition. But it was an impressive enough feat to earn a few "Sugoi!" (*Amazing!*) from my Japanese colleagues, and that's not a word they dole out for trivial matters.

We — Deb, our French friends Mostafa and Severine, and I — started our climb at the fifth station on the Subashiri route. Our goal was to be on the summit to see the sunrise. We would climb through the night. We shared bowls of hot udon noodles and salmon bento boxes, and started the ascent around 7 pm.

We had barely gone a few steps when we heard a thunderous whomp. But thunder and lightening didn't make sense because the sky was clear. Uh-oh. Maybe Fuji-san was growling. It is a volcano after all, albeit one with a low risk of eruption. It last blew its top over 300 years ago. A short while later, another whomp. No, it wasn't coming from inside the mountain, but from down in the valley. We came to the conclusion that we were hearing explosions. Perhaps North Korea was lobbing a few missiles at our heads, but more likely it was something less sinister. We decided to press on with the motto "Leave the wounded behind," just in case.

It took about two hours to reach the next station. The "local management" invited us in. They sipped sake, while we warmed ourselves with tea and hot chocolate. We had a lively conversation in broken Japanese and English, the highlight of which was comparing animal noises. I discovered that there is a difference between how French, Japanese and Canadians make animal sounds. The wild boar living on the mountain say *groin groin* in French, *oink oink* in English and *boo boo* in Japanese.

Back on the trail, Mother Nature gave way to the concerns of nature's call. High above the tree line, there was lava rock and not much else to hide behind when one had to go.

"Are there any toilets ahead?" asked Deb, earnestly.

"Toilet wa everywhere," I said in my best pidgin Japanese, sweeping my hand across the mountain. Mostafa snickered, but Deb and Severine gave me scornful glances, completely unimpressed with my juvenile boys-pee-standing-up humour.

It took about two hours to reach the next hut. The proprietors had closed for the evening and were not offering hot tea or anything else, except an admonition to be quiet. Perhaps they had been warned about the animal noises. We and a dozen other hikers shivered in the cold for a couple of hours. It was midnight and 3 degrees Celsius.

The Pocari Sweat vending machine cast a glow around us. Pocari Sweat is a Japanese sports drink that promises to fight dehydration by replacing lost fluids and minerals. The Evil Glenn loved the name. I imagined every can containing 500 ml of Mr. Pocari's perspiration. Yummy.

We didn't talk much. Occasionally, someone would do jumping jacks to stave off the cold. A yawn inevitably set off a violent shudder. All of us dozed sitting upright. I found myself thinking about Wayne Johnston's novel *The Navigator of New York*. One of the main characters had his trek to the North Pole doubted. Frederick Cook was held up to public scorn and called a charlatan. Eventually the unbelievers outnumbered the believers. Even his most ardent supporters at the Danish Royal Geographical Society began to wonder if he had made it. All of which made me ask myself, If I reach the top how can I prove it to the doubters? A colleague of Cook consoled him (and me) with the assurance that, "The word of a gentleman explorer has always been sufficient proof."

The sake guys had told us that the sun would pop up over the horizon at 5:30. Starting too soon would mean an even colder wait on the summit, famous for its bone-chilling winds. We also wanted to acclimatize. Mt. Fuji is tall enough to cause altitude sickness. Severine's husband had clambered up the mountain previously and then spent most of his time at the top on all fours, retching. We didn't want to repeat his experience. We estimated we were three hours from the summit. We started the final leg at 2 am.

Whatever combination of layers I wore was always the wrong one. It was a rigorous climb and I generated plenty of body heat. I'd strip off the jacket and sweater, only to whip them back on whenever we rested.

We looked like Cape Breton coal miners. Whenever I glanced back, all I could see were headlamps bobbing up and down in the black. The only sound was the jingling of bells attached to walking sticks.

The sky was completely clear, the by-product of a typhoon miles offshore. It had blown every cloud away. Never had I seen so many stars, so clearly. Orion jumped out of the constellations. "It's never been more beautiful," I declared.

By 5 am the first traces of light were on the horizon. We were too tired and the air too thin to make a dash to the top. When we were about 100 metres from the summit, the sky turned red. The Japanese describe it as, "God is coming." We plopped ourselves down and watched the perfect sunrise. We could see forever.

The sunlight revealed the source of the explosions we heard earlier. They were from a quarry. Puffs of dust drifted below. North Korea's threats had been proven empty yet again.

We zigzagged to the top and ate breakfast on the summit: 3776 metres high. Our fits-and-starts climb had taken eight hours of actual walking. We were all exhausted and exhilarated. We reached up and touched the sky. And remember, the word of a gentleman explorer has always been sufficient proof.

"I want you to clamp down on this," said my dentist as she slipped an impression tray into my mouth. The plan was to turn the impressions of my teeth into clay models, exact duplicates of my upper and lower teeth. From those clay models they would make custom-fit dental trays. They resemble the mouth guards that hockey players wear.

I wasn't looking to protect myself from errant pucks; I needed protection from dry mouth. The radiation treatment offered in Toronto might spare my salivary glands and then again it might not. Without saliva I would be more susceptible to cavities, rampant cavities in fact. Spit helps keep harmful bacteria in check. Once radiation started, the only sure way to stop my teeth from rotting out was to coat them in fluoride gel every night for five minutes. Toothpaste alone wouldn't do it. The dental trays would spread the fluoride gel to every nook and cranny in my teeth. The extra fluoride would give the enamel a fighting chance.

All I could think about was Dad and his false teeth. He'd dutifully clean them every night and sit them in a glass of water by his bed. I remember endless discussions between Dad and his friends about which adhesive was best for sticking the teeth to the gums. Among Dad's generation dentures were common; complaints about them were common too.

If only Dad were alive. We'd be able to complain together.

September 17 was a day of accomplishment and regret. Accomplishment because I went back to work. My throat had healed to the point where I couldn't justify staying off another day. Besides, two weeks of moping around the house was long enough. I had regret that Monday, too, because Premier Danny Williams called an election, and just as I predicted, the aliens in my body would prevent me from seeing the campaign through. I was expecting a call from Toronto any day.

That night I watched my colleague Doug Greer cover the Liberal campaign from Bay Roberts. Doug had rolled out of St. John's on the Liberal bus. My cancer-induced loss was his gain. I was envious. My assignment that day was to report on fires in two different schools. No rallies or rides through gorgeous scenery for me. I would have to be content with watching the election as a spectator in the back rows.

I was stunned and couldn't believe what I was reading. Earlier that morning I had picked up copies of my medical records from the cancer clinic. I thought it would be prudent to have the clinical notes, as well as the surgical and pathology reports. Toronto might ask me a question that I couldn't answer.

The source of my dumbfounded reaction was a document with the letterhead *Department of Defense, Armed Forces Institute of Pathology, Washington, D.C.* The official seal was there too, a bald eagle clutching three arrows in its talons. These were the folks who discovered my cancer in the first place. They wrote:

> *Surprisingly, we found a focus of metastatic undifferentiated carcinoma in a small (lymph) node ... no doubt about the diagnosis .... The primary (cancer) still might be ... a poorly differentiated tonsillar carcinoma.*

Tonsil cancer! The doctors in Washington had screamed it out loud from the word go. Incredibly to me, they did it only by looking at microscope slides produced from the lump in my neck. I didn't realize until that moment how insightful their report was. No one told me. I wrongly assumed that Washington had made general statements about my cancer with no precise location.

My God, how good are they at their jobs? The doctors in St. John's said I was cancer-free, that there was nothing sinister in my body. What an incredible gap between the two sets of doctors. How could the Americans be so superb, while the Newfoundland pathologist missed it by a country mile? I was flabbergasted.

I stumbled across an amazing revelation while at my family doctor's clinic. I had a minor ailment and no appointment, but as soon as I mentioned cancer I went to the head of the line. Whoa!

The light that struck Saul on the road to Damascus couldn't have been any brighter than the one that struck me. The heavenly voice said, "Play the cancer card, Glenn, whenever possible."

This was going to be so much better than, "I'm recovering from minor surgery." I couldn't wait to try it out on Deb.

I think my black humour rubbed off on my father-in-law. A friend of Jim's asked him why he was taking so long to build his new house. Jim is a gifted carpenter who specializes in window construction. Need a double-sash wooden window with a curved top to match those already in a 100-year-old house? Jim can make it. In ordinary times, building a house was no problem for him.

Jim told his friend that he was distracted because there were five cases of cancer in the family. He said, "We're a very competitive bunch. We don't like to see anyone get ahead."

I guess I was more competitive than I thought and I'd be taking that competitiveness to Toronto. Dr. Norman's secret handshake had worked. Princess Margaret Hospital invited me for an assessment. I was bound for Toronto the Good with Cancer the Bad.

Toronto

Like so many Newfoundlanders before me, I was headed to Toronto with a one-way ticket. Heaven only knew how long I'd be there. After my assessment Princess Margaret Hospital could send me home for a few weeks or start my treatment the following Monday. My schedule was not my own. I arrived in Toronto for a date with destiny.

The taxi dropped me off outside the main door of Princess Margaret Hospital. It's a towering building on Toronto's University Avenue. I was in the heart of a medical village. There were three other hospitals within a stone's throw. I had arrived in the big leagues.

Princess Margaret proclaims that it's the only facility in Canada devoted exclusively to cancer research, treatment and education. It treated its first cancer patient in 1958, the year I was born. Since then, Princess Margaret has turned cancer treatment into a volume business. It has seventeen radiation machines. I got to know one rather intimately.

Deb had to stay in St. John's because of work commitments. My cousin Ann drove down from Hamilton to be with me. We hugged and kissed in the middle of the atrium. She didn't want me to be alone. I was very grateful.

We made our way to the Wharton Head and Neck Centre. Imagine, a whole clinic dedicated to head and neck cancers, operating five days a week. Suddenly I didn't feel unique. Somebody in that room probably had tonsil cancer too.

The night before, I dreamt about arriving at the clinic. A doctor entered the examination room and I introduced myself. He didn't return the courtesy and curtly said, "Oh, we don't bother with such things here." Even for Toronto that was cold.

Back in the real world, Ann and I were swapping family gossip as we waited for Dr. John Waldron, the radiation oncologist assigned to me. A man came in. I stood up, shook his hand and introduced Ann and myself.

"I'm Dr. Wasim Phoplunkar," he said in a thick Indian accent.

"I'm sorry, what was that?"

"I'm Dr. Wasim Phoplunkar."

"I'm sorry, but I still didn't catch it."

"I'm Dr. Wasim Phoplunkar."

"Would you please write that down?" Perhaps we all would have been better off if he had said, "Oh, we don't bother with such things here."

Dr. Phoplunkar explained that he was a fellow in the hospital, which is a doctor studying a subspecialty. Dr. Waldron would join us in a few minutes.

The first order of business was to push a fibre optic hose up my nose. Yet another doctor who made a beeline for the flexible scope. What was it about my nasal cavity and throat that they were all dying to see? Perhaps it was some hazing ritual for tonsil cancer patients. Better than a paddling, I suppose. Dr. Phoplunkar said everything was normal. Soon there was a snowstorm of paper flying between us. Not all my medical records had arrived from St. John's. Good thing I had copies.

Dr. Waldron came in and after the pleasantries he reached for the flexible scope and said, "Let's have a look."

I wanted to scream, "Enough already with the rubber hose

up the nose shtick. The novelty has worn off." Dr. Waldron would be doctor number four exploring that nether region. Did the entire lot of them have a misspent youth listening to the Cheech and Chong routine "Up His Nose"?

"Can you put that on the TV?" asked Ann.

"Sure can," said Dr. Waldron. It was a *Star Trek* moment. Ann and I would boldly go where we hadn't gone before.

The back of the tongue is a scary sight. It's potholed, far worse than any St. John's street. The highlight of the tour was my voice box. The TV monitor made it twenty inches wide. The little flaps changed shape as I said hello. There was healthy-looking pink flesh wherever the camera turned. It was fascinating, as Mr. Spock would say. Oh, for the record, unlike the ne'er-do-well on the Cheech and Chong album, there were no silver dollars up *my* nose.

"How was McGill?" I asked Dr. Waldron.

"Ah, you've been checking my CV."

I explained that my Grandfather Forbes was a doctor in Bonavista and he trained at McGill. Dr. Waldron complained that he didn't get to enjoy the city during the two years he was there because all he did was study. Such a shame. Montreal is a wonderful city.

Dr. Waldron told me that they intended to recheck the pathology. "Especially since it's from Newfoundland," he said. "Just kidding. We do this with every new patient, even ones from hospitals in Ontario." I wasn't the least bit slighted. Given the fact that the Newfoundland pathologist had missed the cancer in my neck lump in the first place, I welcomed a second opinion on that and the tonsil cancer.

Dr. Waldron was as definite about the need for radiation treatment as the radiation oncologist in St. John's. "A surgeon can only take what he can see with his eyes. He can't see the microscopic. The cancer could have sent out tentacles. There can be a million cancer cells on the head of a pin."

Dr. Waldron put my chances for a cure at 85 per cent. It was only 5 fewer percentage points than Dr. Norman in St. John's had given me, but I wanted them back. Doctors! Will they ever agree? Still, 85 per cent was good odds. No guarantees of course, just his best guess, but his message was one of hope.

It was hard to reconcile how healthy I felt that day with the danger I might be in. I told Dr. Waldron, "On Saturday I ran two and a half miles. I split wood by swinging an axe for three hours. And I put up the storm windows on my house. Yet I have, or had, cancer. I never know what tense to use."

We spent a fair bit of time chatting about the side effects of radiation and how to mitigate them. Some were familiar, like dry mouth, damaged taste buds and weeping skin around my neck. Others were brand new, such as the loss of hair on the back of my neck. I hadn't really considered it before but the body doesn't stop radiation. If it goes in, it must come out. Radiation kills fast growing cells like cancer and hair. The back of my neck might get a blotchy look, perhaps matching the blotchy look in my beard.

There was an unexpected and unsettling development. It made the hair on my yet-to-be-irradiated neck stand up. Dr. Waldron suggested that I might need chemotherapy in addition to radiation. No one had mentioned this before.

In the short term, I would be much sicker. The chemo drug of choice was cisplatin — a drug with an awful reputation. Vomiting and nausea are among its ghastly side effects. Having chemo would lengthen my radiation treatment from five weeks to seven. My body wouldn't be able to tolerate the higher radiation dosage of the five-week program.

I would likely suffer dramatic and permanent hearing loss, so profound that I would need hearing aids. Also eating, in all probability, would be impossible. They would insert a feeding tube directly into my stomach. It had to be done before the dual treatment started. They had seen patients in the past wait too long to have the tube inserted. Those patients lost worrisome amounts of weight. Dr. Waldron had arranged for me to see a medical oncologist and he'd accept whatever decision we made.

78

Dr. Waldron wasn't completely Dr. Grim. On the upside, he held out the possibility of zapping only one side of my neck. He'd decide after reviewing all the medical reports.

We said our goodbyes and Dr. Waldron was almost out the door when he turned and said, "If you're a wine connoisseur, you might want to drink the Bordeaux now." Sage advice. I vowed to take a few vintage bottles off the rack when I got home.

Being "sick" did have its advantages. Once Dr. Waldron was finished with me, I was free to have fun for a few days. Ann carted me back to Hamilton for supper with her husband Kurt. It was so hot and humid that all he could bear to prepare were tomato and bacon sandwiches.

"They're so good I want the recipe," I said with a mocking tone. Kurt took the jab in good humour.

My cousin Lynn and her husband Norm joined us the following evening. Lynn arrived with family heirlooms and stories that I had never heard before. She had a striking silver locket with the name Ruby on the front. Inside were a lock of Ruby's hair and a photo. Ruby's eyes were closed and it looked as though she was lying down. I had seen this kind of picture before. It was a death photo. This was Ruby laid out at her wake. It sounds morbid, but such photos were common in the 1800s and early 1900s. They were considered a dignified remembrance of a loved one.

The story goes that Ruby died when other children buried her in sand. Her chest collapsed and she couldn't breathe. Ruby was my Grandmother Forbes' sister. I suspect my grandmother carried that locket until the day she died. Lynn got it from Aunt Viv, my mother's sister.

Lynn also had photographs of my mother as a little girl. Kathleen Forbes she was then. Mom and her siblings were on a camping trip in the woods, a few miles from their hometown of Bonavista. They're all dead now, except for Aunt Viv. But in those 1920s photos, they were gleeful kids camping with their mom and dad in a canvas tent that had no floor and was propped up with limbed-out trees. I had forgotten my mother's smile.

Cancer killed Mom. I was reminded of it every time I met a new doctor. They all wanted to know my family's medical history, particularly the cases of cancer. Mom contracted breast cancer in 1972 and brain cancer in 1975. She was just fifty-nine when she died. I was seventeen and in my last year of high school.

I accepted that the doctors needed to know this stuff, but it brought me back to a painful time nevertheless. I was in the hospital room when she took her last breath. It was blessed relief because she suffered terribly at the end. That kind of memory never fades. It was good to put a memory of the smiling little girl in the photos alongside it.

My sweet cousin Ann is a dragon lady. And I mean that in the nicest possible way. She coaches a dragon boat team and she invited Lynn and me to watch their last practice of the season. Everyone in the boat had stared down death and was full of life. They were all breast cancer survivors.

If laughter alone could cure cancer then this crowd would never have to worry again. One woman had us howling by telling the bad luck story behind her hobble. She couldn't bend her big toe because two fighting squirrels tumbled over her foot and drove a claw into a tendon. Her foot would probably require surgery.

The crew was a couple of paddlers short, so at the last minute Lynn and I were ordered into the dragon boat. This was a fun practice, but the women didn't want us making a mess of their routine. We got a quick lesson about posture and following the stroke in front of us. We were in the middle section of the boat: six paddlers affectionately dubbed "engine room." It was full steam ahead out into Hamilton Harbour.

Everyone was in good spirits. Among our crew was a doctor specializing in sports medicine. The women offered to take him out for a spin to show him the potential injuries paddlers might one day bring into his office. Ann says doctors often dismiss their injuries because they think the women are lily-dipping.

We were put through our paces. A fifteen-minute warm-up paddle, standing starts, men only, women only, sprints. No lily-dippers here. There were jokes about the fast stroke causing a stroke. It was exhausting.

"What a bitch!" I muttered to the delight of the other paddlers.

"What was that?" My darling cousin raised three kids so she has the knack of catching remarks said under the breath.

"I have a bad itch," I yelled back.

"Good recovery," someone whispered behind me.

"Engine room," shouted Ann. "On your own."

When will I learn to keep my big mouth shut? It seemed like an eternity before another section of the boat was ordered to paddle. Still, no one seemed to mind. If cancer didn't kill them, a vengeful coach beating up on her cousin certainly wouldn't.

Norm and I went for a jog around Hamilton's Bayfront Park. As we trotted around the marina and curved boardwalks, we swapped war stories. To me, Norm's experience was the epitome of good medicine. He had what I wanted, but wouldn't get.

Norm used to have a heart condition. Years earlier, the electrical impulses in his heart were sometimes random and chaotic. His heart could go into uncontrolled fluttering with no warning. The problem had become more debilitating over time. At first, Norm had to be wary of too much exercise, but later, even something sedentary like sitting at his desk could cause an episode. His doctors decided to cauterize the problem section of his heart. The operation was wildly successful. Jogging, biking, sailing — now there was no activity that Norm had to be afraid of.

I confessed that I was envious. Medical intervention had dramatically improved his quality of life. Medical intervention would do the opposite for me. Norm was sick; the doctors made him healthy. I was healthy; the doctors were going to make me sick. Worse than that, I'd never be as good after they were done with me, as I was that day jogging with Norm. Telling my doctors, "Why can't you be like Norm's doctors?" didn't strike me as a very mature approach, but the thought crossed my mind.

My sister Judy once said, "I never knew how to laugh until I had cancer." Judy was a prodigious smoker and she paid the price. Cancer showed up in her right lung. A surgeon saved her life by cutting out the top third of the lung. Several years later, Judy was diagnosed with a malignant brain tumour. Tests proved that the cancer on her brain had migrated from the cancer in her lung. Again, a surgeon saved Judy's life.

There was nothing funny of course in any of the operating room drama. Judy found humour during her radiation therapy afterwards, more specifically, the lodge where she stayed while getting treatment in Hamilton. Whenever I spoke to her on the phone I could hear convulsions of laughter in the background. I swear Judy and those other patients laughed themselves back to good health.

Judy was just an hour's drive away. I decided to make a quick visit to Kitchener. She was living in a retirement home because she couldn't keep her balance. Even though Judy used a walker she was prone to falling, and living on her own was too danger-ous. Moving into Trinity Village was actually a fortunate turn of events. Judy rediscovered romance in the home. She met a man and was anxious for me to meet him.

Judy and Larry were smitten with each other. Judy had told me the story of their first kiss. Larry had escorted her back to her room and made his move. He pulled Judy close. What he didn't realize was that he was pressing against her alarm necklace. Buzzers were going off down the hall at the nursing station. Judy's phone rang and a concerned voice asked, "Mrs. Dyke, are you all right? Is everything okay?" Judy turned beet-red and was completely flustered. Never had a first kiss been so interrupted.

Larry doted on my sister. All three of us shared a long walk and dinner together. Judy never looked happier. When we were alone Larry leaned in to tell me, "We haven't had sex yet, but I have a birthday before Halloween." There was hope in his eyes. When I told Judy later she smiled and said, "Trick or treat."

Cancer tried twice to kill Judy. Thankfully, it failed twice. Yes, cancer robbed her of some of her vitality. But it failed to steal her sense of humour or her desire to feel love, or lust, for that matter. It was an unspoken lecture. Suck it up, Glenn. There's lots more living to be done.

Five minutes inside Princess Margaret Hospital Lodge and I was reminded that I had no right to feel sorry for myself. I saw a woman wearing a bandage where her nose should be. A young man struggled with a walker. An older man had a skin graft on his face right over one eye. There were assorted people carrying pumps and wheeling intravenous bags around. They all looked far worse off than I did. There, but for the grace of God, go I.

Princess Margaret Hospital Lodge would be my home for the next couple of nights. Dr. Waldron had arranged a sprinkling of tests and examinations. The lodge was a sanctuary to dozens of people like me, people on the verge of cancer treatment or in the full throes of it.

Nurse Terry had to write up my medical file before giving me a tour. She inquired about the possibility of my having a feeding tube. I'm not sure why but the prospect of a feeding tube gave me the cold shivers, even more than the prospect of radiation.

The gastrostomy entailed having a tube with a light on the end pushed down my throat into my stomach. The light would shine through the abdominal wall, essentially telling the doctor to cut here. He'd make a small incision and stick in the feeding tube. All of this would be done while I was awake.

I explained that the necessity of a feeding tube had yet to be determined and would only happen if I had chemo as well as radiation. Nurse Terry thought I should consider one no matter what the circumstances. "The feeding tube is your friend. It gives you water, food and medication." Maybe so, but all I could think about was gagging down a scope, and a hole in my stomach.

Nurse Terry guided me around the lodge. There is a computer room, laundry room, a piano lounge, a cafeteria and beds for over 100 people. Nurses are on duty 24 hours a day.

"This place works really well. No doctors," she said quietly.

Nurse Terry offered insight on the neighbours as we strolled through the corridors. "Church Street is the centre of the gay community and some of the girls are not girls, even if they look like girls. And there are lots of prostitutes in the area." Sounded like I was in a fun neighbourhood.

We stepped outside into a lovely courtyard. "Feel free to use this whenever you want. The smokers are down at the far end."

"You're kidding."

"It's a very stressful time for people. We try not to preach. We encourage them to cut down."

I was thankful that, unlike the smokers, I didn't have to fight two demons at once.

"Excuse me," said the Asian man in halting English, "do you know where to find the Art Gallery of Ontario?"

What luck! I did know where the Art Gallery of Ontario was. I had walked past it only thirty seconds before. It was undergoing a massive renovation and partially hidden behind scaffolding and bright blue tarps. I was just about to play the role of the friendly local and point towards the AGO when I noticed Japanese characters on their city map.

"Sumimasen, Nihon-jin desu ka?" I asked. *Excuse me, are you Japanese?*

"Hai!" said Mrs. Tourist. *Yes!*

Mr. Tourist was having none of this speaking Japanese in Toronto nonsense. "The art gallery, do you know where it is?"

I pointed at the monstrous building on the other side of Dundas Street and said, "Asoko desu." *Over there, that place.*

Mr. Tourist still refused to speak to me in Japanese. "The blue one?"

"Hai." *Yes.*

"Domo arigato," said Mrs. Tourist, bowing slightly. *Thank you.*

"Do itashimashite," I replied, bowing slightly as well. *You're welcome.*

Inoue-san would have been proud. She was my Japanese teacher, my sensei. If my Japanese ever grated her ear, she never showed it. Inoue-san was the grandmotherly type and her encouragement never faltered. "Oh, you good student." She said it in such a way that I felt like I was four and was being patted on the head for having just learned how to tie my shoes. She was innocently funny. She always used Yogi Berra-isms like, "It's easy, but difficult" and "It's the same, but different."

Whenever I let her praise balloon my head, someone would take a needle and prick it. One night in Tokyo I was chatting with a bar owner and he asked me, in English, where I lived. I answered in Japanese.

"Shibuya-ku no, Nishihara-ni sunde imasu." *I live in the Nishihara district of Shibuya.*

He shook his head. "Ahh, my English is not so good."

The unintentional put-downs didn't end there. At work there was a Kando-san and a Kondo-san. You would think that a budding linguist, who had conquered not one but two Japanese alphabets, could clearly enunciate the ka and the ko sounds. Apparently not. No matter which name I called out, both heads snapped around. Having been falsely summoned one too many times, Saori Kando decided to give me an impromptu lesson in pronunciation.

"Kando," she said rounding her lips.

"Kando," I replied, convinced I was saying it perfectly.

"No, it's Kando."

"Kando."

She grimaced. "Kando," with emphasis on the ka.

"Kando."

She had an exasperated look, as if to ask, "How in heaven's name can you not get it?" There was no, "Oh, you good student." Clearly, I did not have the nuance of a native speaker. The next day she arrived at my desk and announced to the amusement of everyone around, "I am Saori Kando." The Tanaka-san twins had big smiles. They weren't really twins at all, but that's a story for another day.

I thought later, perhaps it wasn't the quality of my Japanese that prompted Mr. Tourist not to respond in kind. He might have simply wanted to practice his English.

I was reminded of an incident at Yasukuni Shrine. Yasukuni is the most controversial piece of real estate in all of Japan. It's a memorial to Japan's war dead. Among the souls enshrined there are fourteen convicted war criminals. I went on August 15, the anniversary of Japan's surrender in the Second World War, though proud Japanese simply refer to it as the day the war stopped. I was in a crowd of thousands, including ultra-nationalists dressed in military-like uniforms.

I saw a man making a beeline towards me. I doubted he was a right-wing extremist. His fashion sense was a dead giveaway. His waistband was closer to his armpits than his hips. I was spared a lecture on how America lured Japan into bombing Pearl Harbor.

"What country are you from?"

"Kanada jin desu," I answered, being polite I thought. *I'm Canadian.*

"Speak English, I want to practice. Canada, ah yes, ten provinces. British Columbia, Alberta, Saskatchewan …"

Incredible! I had stumbled across the only man in Japan who had devoured the *Canadian Encyclopedia* and he was about to recite it all back to me.

"What province are you from?

"Newfoundland."

"Ah, it was once a country and joined Canada in 1948, no, 1949."

He wasn't so much interested in hearing me speak English as hearing himself speak English. It was the longest five-minute "conversation" I ever had.

It seems to me that the Japanese have a love/hate relationship with English. Never have so many studied so much to master so little. The Evil Glenn was thankful for it really. If Japanese universally spoke good English, the mystifying English concoctions that adorn packaging and buildings throughout Japan would not have been there to entertain me. Where else can you walk past the Crossbred Kitchen café and discover that the Heartbrake Killers are playing at the Heavy Sick bar? English is the language of marketing in Japan. It's cool and doesn't have to make sense because it is simply ornamental.

I put such cynicism aside, however, when I signed on to teach my native tongue to the schoolgirls at Yakumo Academy. The ninth grade girls in their blue uniforms couldn't have been more earnest about learning the language. This was their annual English fun fair. A full Saturday morning devoted to practising English with dozens of native speakers.

We played tongue twisters (How much wood would a woodchuck chuck, if a woodchuck could chuck wood?) and Simon Says. Some of the girls were painfully shy about speaking English, while others were gung ho.

They all had a list of questions: How long have you been in Japan? What country do you come from? What is your favourite Japanese food? Can you use chopsticks? Completely innocuous questions, and not original. I had heard them dozens of times before, usually during dead-end conversations in bars. The conversation invariably ground to a halt whenever the list of questions ran out.

One student asked, "Are you from Pakistan?" I'm not sure what list she was reading from. Many asked, "What's your favourite animal?" How convenient that I had brought a prop with me — a photo of a caribou.

Now the Evil Glenn would have said, "Ya, it's a beauty. I shot one just like it with a Thirty-Aught-Six, gutted it right away, sawed it in four pieces, cut out the heart, and ate it with some fava beans and a nice Chianti." But the image of screaming girls running from the room in full panic prevented me from spinning that yarn.

I went with the more wholesome, "What does this remind you of?"

"Reindeer," someone would inevitably muster the courage to say.

"Yes, Santa's reindeer. We have them where I live in Canada."

I charmed them with stories of caribou, whales and icebergs, and never let on that they were sitting next to the Hannibal Lector of the Newfoundland barrens.

The Mask

My time in Toronto was all a little surreal. Never more so than when they cast my immobilization mask. I was lying on a CT scan table. The technicians explained that the mask would bolt me to the radiation table during treatment. Moving around when you're being zapped is not recommended.

The mask started out as a flat plastic mesh stretched across a C-shaped frame. It resembled a bucksaw. They first put the mesh in a hot water bath to make it soft and malleable. Next, they held the frame over my nose and then pushed it down over my face, head, neck and shoulders, stretching the mesh right to the table. They screwed the frame down and covered it with cool towels to make it harden.

"Swallow a few times," she said. "It loosens the area around the Adam's apple." I had to lie perfectly still for five minutes.

"You're tolerating it well," she said. "So I'll leave it there a while longer. It will be better for you." All I could do was grunt approval and be thankful for living today. Years ago they used to make the mask out of plaster.

The technicians were pleased with their handiwork. The mask was sculpted perfectly to my upper physique. Soon I would wear it for about fifteen minutes a day, five days a week, for five weeks.

It was strange looking at myself, or what was supposed to be me. I had to admit there was a resemblance. I thought of the ghoulish fun I could have petrifying the trick-or-treaters next Halloween. Actor Jim Carrey's mask turned him into a diabolically funny man. I was uneasy about what my mask would turn me into.

"My dentist says I should ignore everything you say, if you contradict her," I jokingly said to Dr. Maxymiw.

"Really. And how many head and neck patients has she seen?" Dr. Walter Maxymiw was Chief of Dentistry at Princess Margaret Hospital, and his tone told me that he didn't appreciate my attempt at humour.

"I think I'm the only one," I said sheepishly.

"Well, I've seen hundreds."

"Dr. Roberts is my sister-in-law," I said, hoping the family connection would explain the remark and soften him up. It seemed to work.

Even though Sarah had given me a thorough check-up before my trip to Toronto, Princess Margaret had its own dentists, thank you very much. Dr. Maxymiw was looking for infections and cavities, and most importantly, he was checking for teeth that would have to be pulled.

Bone exposed to high levels of radiation undergoes irreversible damage. The blood vessels narrow; the bone essentially dies. If a tooth has to be extracted, it's best done before radiation because the gum won't heal properly afterwards.

"Your sister-in-law does good work." Dr. Maxymiw didn't see any dental problems. "You know, years ago we used to pull all the teeth before radiation."

That prospect made me shudder. Once again I thought of Dad and his false teeth. Without them he couldn't speak properly. Thank God, pulling teeth was no longer the accepted dental practice.

Dr. Maxymiw wanted to see the dental trays that Sarah had

cast the next time I came in for a check-up. That would be half-way through the radiation treatment.

"Will I have to wear them for the rest of my life?"

"Maybe. It depends on how well your saliva recovers."

When you have dry mouth, the cavity-producing bacteria outnumber the good bacteria.

Dr. Maxymiw wanted a baseline measurement of my saliva output. I was a phenomenal drooler when asleep. But "patient once soaked T-shirt while dozing upright on the Newfoundland ferry" wasn't really a medical description. Dr. Maxymiw had a simple and accurate test to measure saliva.

He used a paper strip that was first developed to test for eye dryness. It was calibrated in millimetres and impregnated with blue dye. Dr. Maxymiw held the strip under my tongue. As the saliva pooled, the blue dye revealed itself and travelled up the strip. The test was supposed to last three minutes, with the amount being recorded at one-, two- and three-minute intervals. But my salivary glands acted like a broken water main. They were pumping so much spit that Dr. Maxymiw gave up after a minute and a half, and told his assistant to record the maximum amount — about two tablespoons in three minutes. No wonder my pillow was always wet in the morning. I drooled like Homer Simpson dreaming of pork chops. How depressing to think that I was going to lose almost all of it.

The dentist's chair wasn't the end of the medical poking and prod-ding. Dr. Waldron had ordered a CT scan on my chest, blood tests and a hearing test. I joked with the audiologist that according to my wife, I'm already deaf because I never hear a word she says.

"Oh, we never listen to the wives," she said. "They tend not to be very accurate."

Chemotherapy is known to cause temporary or permanent damage to the inner ear, but the side effects from radiation aren't as well documented. The audiologist gave me a brochure that listed hearing loss, ringing in the ears, more earwax and increased pressure in the ears as possible side effects.

The audiologist discovered that I had lost some hearing in the upper range of my left ear, but I was nowhere near as deaf as Deb thought. With that, I was free to escape the clutches of the cancer clinic until the next week.

My cousin Lynn and I had planned a road trip to Ottawa. Our quest was to see Aunt Viv, sister to my mom and sister to Lynn's dad. Aunt Viv had recently moved into a retirement home and was having extended confusion spells. She smiled widely when we walked into her apartment.

"Come in, dear, come in." Even though she never called us by name, there was recognition in her eyes. She teetered a little on her feet. "The town drunk," she said. She laughed at her own unsteadiness. Still, she was game to give us a tour of the home. We stayed close to her and her walker.

Aunt Viv was eighty-nine and fading. "This is where the kids come to make things," she said, as she led us into the craft room. There were no kids of course. The residents, seniors all, were the only people who made anything in that room. The hair salon seemed foreign to her, but she had been there several times before. Aunt Viv was rediscovering the same things every day.

What a contrast to the Aunt Viv who worked in a top-secret cartography office during World War II. Once, a map went missing, and for a time Aunt Viv was a prime suspect. Then she remembered a man who had been there days before, asking a lot of questions that he shouldn't have been asking. Eventually, the investigators discovered that he was the thief. Aunt Viv passed him in a hallway on the way to his court martial. She hauled off and decked him. The punch got Aunt Viv a court martial of her own. The officer in charge could barely contain his delight at handing out the minimum punishment possible, confining her to barracks for a day. My Aunt Viv. Don't get on her wrong side.

I never mentioned my cancer to Aunt Viv. No good could come of it. I don't think she would have understood, but if she had, I ran the risk of upsetting her needlessly. Hiding my illness seemed the right thing to do.

Afterwards, Lynn and I had lunch downtown and strolled around the ByWard Market. I spied a kiosk selling maple syrup cookies, and their sign had Japanese characters, presumably for all the Japanese tourists who land in Ottawa. I dragged Lynn over, mostly to show off and prove that I could actually read the language.

"This is kukkii, cookie."

"You can speak Japanese?" asked the young Japanese woman behind the counter.

"Nihongo ga sukoshi wakarimasu." *I understand a little Japanese.*

We had a chat in Japanese about my time in her home country. She asked simple questions and I gave simple answers. I liberally drew from the seventy or so Japanese stock phrases that I had mastered. Lynn was very impressed. Mission accomplished.

Learning the ABCs of Japanese wasn't easy for me. The Japanese have three alphabets, and I conquered only two. The hardest part was getting the symbols to stick in my brain. Most of them don't look anything like our letters, except several that resemble "n." I was forgetting them as fast as I looked at them. So, I started playing word association. I stared at a symbol until it reminded me of something or someone. For example, ke is pronounced Kay — my mother's name. That particular symbol has a cross in it. Mom was a church lady, so I dubbed that one "Kay's cross." I associated symbols with animals, English phrases, and parts of the body — anything to help me remember. I practised writing them over and over. Finally, they sunk in.

As I walked around Tokyo in the early months, I read signs out loud. I didn't have a clue what the words meant, but I could pronounce them. My first eureka moment came when I passed a fabric shop and read ki-mo-no, kimono. I wanted to jump and yell, "I know what that is!" But boisterous displays are frowned on in Japan, so I said it only to myself.

Linguistic swagger had its perils though. I stood by one big sign on a promenade and brazenly read the symbols out loud several times, correcting mistakes as I went along. After finishing, I took one step past the sign and discovered a bewildered-looking homeless man lying on a park bench. God only knows what he thought. Probably, Those crazy foreigners!

Lynn and I continued our meandering and walked into a shop that sold curios from Indonesia. They had a carving called a whispering ghost. A cardboard note said if I whispered a wish into its ear, the wish would come true.

I moved on and spied a bin of wooden penis bottle openers. As tacky as they were, I flippantly thought maybe I should get one of these for Deb; after all, it might be the only erect penis she'd see for a couple of months. It's not that I had trouble in that department. I was thinking that with the physical changes my body was about to undergo, coupled with the stress of the radiation, that would, well, you know, make it difficult to … um … LOOK, IT'S NONE OF YOUR DAMN BUSINESS.

I went back to the whispering ghost, leaned into an ear and said softly, "No side effects."

That night I dreamt that I was sitting at my desk in the CBC newsroom in St. John's. One of *Here & Now*'s hosts, Jonathan Crowe, strolled over.

"What's the headline, Glenn?"

I glanced up. "I'm not going to die."

Jonathan turned on his heels and walked away. In one way, the dream was frighteningly accurate. Newsroom talk is often truncated. People are up against unforgiving deadlines. They only want the information required for that instant. Make it fast, make it accurate. On the other hand, the dream was completely unfair to Jonathan. He would never behave that callously in real life. I didn't know whether he had any idea about my cancer. I had chosen to tell only two friends at work and I swore them to secrecy. I didn't want my cancer to be water cooler talk. I had told friends and family, and that was enough. I wanted privacy.

It seemed to me that ever since the cancer diagnosis I had had a few days of destiny. Never more so than my last medical appointment at Princess Margaret Hospital before I hopped a flight home. I was scheduled to meet with Dr. Lillian Siu, a medical oncologist. We needed to decide whether I would have chemotherapy on top of radiation. Ann drove down from Hamilton again to be with me during a key appointment.

Dr. Siu walked into the room wearing a bright smile. My first thought was not how lucky I was to be seeing this highly respected doctor, who squeezed me into an already busy day. No, I was thinking, Attractive Asian woman. How stupid! I was there to discuss a critical decision about my treatment and my mind was saying, "She's very good looking." I gave myself a mental slap up the side of the head and started listening very carefully.

I had already learned that medicine is an art form, not an exact science. Dr. Siu only enforced my belief. "This is a matter of philosophy, not medicine," she said. "My job would be so much easier if this were a more advanced cancer. I'd be saying take the chemo, there's no choice."

She first laid out the pros of taking chemo. "You have an aggressive cancer because it's shown a willingness to travel." That was undeniably true. The lump in my neck was cancer pretending to be Columbus, an explorer of new worlds. Cancer cells went from my tonsil to my neck, and could possibly travel the lymph node highway around my body.

I was a healthy forty-nine-year-old and Dr. Siu had no doubt that I could tolerate the treatment, despite the nausea. "You'll be sick. Everyone gets sick except the alcoholics. Nothing makes them sick."

The most important consideration: this would be the one and only time that I could simultaneously have chemo and radiation to my neck, the only time for a one-two punch. The reason: you can irradiate a part of the body only once. Chemo would suppress the cancer cells in between the radiation sessions, allowing the radiation to work better. That's the accepted theory anyway.

"This is the only time to cure with chemo," said Dr. Siu. "If the cancer recurs, surgery is the only curable option."

"So chemo could only keep it in remission?"

"Yes. I can't tell if the cancer cells have spread somewhere else. We don't see it now and we don't want to see it when the treatment is over."

I mused that I and every other cancer patient needed a simple blood test to tell if cancer cells have migrated around the body. Maybe in the future, but it didn't exist when I was in Dr. Siu's office and it still doesn't exist today.

We slid into a discussion of the cons. "Usually chemo gives you an extra 5 to 10 per cent advantage that your cancer won't come back. That's huge. In your case there's less than an extra 5 per cent benefit." She really couldn't be more precise. The medical literature was unclear.

"If you were in the United States, there would be no question here. You would have both. In Canada, we try to be more reflective. I worry about overkill. I can't tell whether it will do any good or not."

The con argument revolved around compounding the radiation's side effects, and piling on new ones, both short and long term. Calling in the heavy artillery would almost certainly leave me with significant and permanent hearing loss. "Ten per cent loss is the norm," said Dr. Siu.

I could also suffer kidney damage, plus persistent numbness and tingling in my hands and feet. Dr. Siu said she once had a patient who was a concert pianist. After just one chemo treatment he had numbness in his fingertips. She stopped the chemo right away. "If I notice dramatic side effects, you're done."

A combination of chemo and radiation would necessitate

my hospitalization one day a week, for seven weeks. They would keep me overnight to make sure that I was properly hydrated.

Dr. Siu asked whether Deb and I were planning children, since chemo can affect fertility. I explained that since I was forty-nine and she was forty-seven, time had really made the decision for us.

"What about impotence?" I asked, with the sudden dread that there are fates worse than dying from cancer. Ann gave me a little eye roll.

Dr. Siu replied, "The machinery will work fine. There just won't be any oil."

Before walking into Dr. Siu's office, the radiation oncologist in St. John's had given me a 90 per cent chance of a cure with radiation alone. The radiation oncologist in Toronto had pegged my chances at 85 per cent. I considered those pretty good odds. I told Dr. Siu, "Radiation will hurt me. Chemo will hurt me even more. I'm thinking about how to limit the hurt."

"Most people sitting across from me only worry about the cure. They say, 'Give me everything you've got.' You're obviously thinking beyond the cure and that's fine. I wonder if I'm spraying pesticide around for no good reason." It was a brilliant analogy.

"This decision is about regrets," she said. Was it ever. Making the wrong choice might invite the cancer back — or leave me with a diminished quality of life for no good reason.

"I wouldn't disagree with you if you said no. I wouldn't be opposed if you said yes. I want to give you every chance I can."

If the chemo did no lasting harm, I could see putting up with the short-term side effects to get those extra percentage points. The worse mouth sores, the feeding tube in my stomach, the nausea and the hair loss. As awful as they sounded, I could endure them for the right reason. But I couldn't see the greater good here. The evidence was less than convincing. At the end of the hour, my mind was almost made up. I needed to talk it over with Deb though. I promised Dr. Siu an answer the next day.

Ann drove me from Dr. Siu's office to the airport. Along the way we reconstructed the conversation and I made notes. Ann and I hugged goodbye knowing that we would see each other again soon. I was welcome to visit them in Hamilton anytime I wanted during my treatment.

I got back to St. John's late and decided to put off my medical chat with Deb until after breakfast the next morning. When my stomach was full and I could think straight, I recited Dr. Siu's opinions. Deb worried that I was fixating on the side effects and not the cure.

"Show me the compelling argument for chemo," I said. "I don't see it." A good night's sleep had convinced me to say no to chemo. I was stopping the hurt at radiation.

"It's your decision; you have to live with it. Just tell me it's the right one."

I hugged her and whispered, "It's the right one."

We embraced for a bit and Deb said, "I'll need a plastic surgeon after this."

"Why?"

"I'm going to be full of wrinkles. Just don't take too long to recover because I'm next in line."

Dr. Siu phoned me that afternoon. I was on the first hole of Bally Haly golf course. It was another surreal moment. I was telling my doctor about a life and death decision between a drive and a chip to the green.

I picked up my ball and walked away from my playing partners.

"Dr. Siu, I appreciate your candour and the way you laid out my options. I'm going to say, No thank you."

"I'm not surprised," she said. "It's a perfectly reasonable decision. If I thought otherwise, I'd be telling you to think about it again."

"Dr. Siu, if I've made the wrong call, it's on my conscience, not yours."

"Let's hope we never meet again," she said.

For the first time since my diagnosis I felt in control. Finally,

I could make the decision. I smashed the ball off the number two tee. It was a lousy drive — a slice into the woods. But I felt good. I was enjoying a game of golf with pleasant company under blue skies with crisp temperatures. If I had known cancer was going to be this much fun, I would have had it sooner.

"I think that's a reasonable decision," said Dr. Waldron. I called him after the golf game and was glad to hear that he also endorsed my unwillingness to accept chemotherapy. Now he was on to the practical matter of designing my radiation treatment.

Dr. Waldron had disappointing news though. After reviewing the pathology reports, he had decided to irradiate both sides of my neck. The salivary gland on the side with my tonsil cancer would get a full dosage, the other side a lower dosage, but one that would still cause unpleasantness. My vocal cords would receive no radiation. That was a blessing at least.

"I'm being cautious." Dr. Waldron believed that the tumour in my neck might have been larger originally. "Your immune system may have knocked it down and reduced the size." The neck tumour had crossed his comfort threshold, and two sides of neck irradiation were better than one in my case.

Just when I thought I had heard it all, Dr. Waldron raised the possibility of a new side effect — cancer caused by the radiation itself. "Usually it's only a possibility in very young patients who have a lifetime to grow the cancer." However, he felt compelled to inform me about the potential danger. Full disclosure is what I wanted and full disclosure is what I got.

I was jogging around Long Pond in St. John's when I saw her. She was rounding the bend ahead of me so I got a good look. She was of Asian descent. I thought of all the wonderful Tokyo moments I witnessed because of jogging.

It may sound pretentious to say, but when I lived in Tokyo I lived in Shangri-la. That was the name written on the brass plaque bolted to my apartment building. My little utopia in Tokyo. And where else but paradise would you see a gorgeous woman in a peach kimono.

That morning outside Shangri-la I looked like a slob — shorts, T-shirt and sweaty. I had just finished a long run in sultry weather. I casually stretched and stole looks from a discreet distance. The woman in the peach kimono was pacing nervously, obviously late for some appointment. She quickly shuffled towards a taxi in her white socks and sandals, only to realize that it wasn't the one she ordered. More fretting. I was stretching some muscles a second or third time, anything not to go inside.

There is sensuality to a kimono because it hides a woman's figure, and yet, it accentuates just the right amount of curvature. It's quintessentially feminine and alluring. Her taxi did arrive eventually and she left to brighten someone else's day.

That moment outside Shangri-la was bliss. Running around Long Pond in St. John's, I angrily realized that there might never be another Shangri-la moment in my life. Cancer might steal the exotic from me. It might make me too sick to pursue the next "Japan." I ran past the Asian jogger and surged up the hills. I ran with vitriol in my heart. And when I finished I looked up at the sky and said, "Fuck you, cancer!"

The Pit

How many times had Steve and I sipped cognac at Christian's Bar? That number might frighten even the most stalwart George Street reprobates. Remy Martin owned our souls on those nights. And we were prepared to give the demon cognac one more chance to enslave us.

Princess Margaret Hospital had called. My radiation therapy would start October 15. The medical brochures warned me to avoid spicy foods and alcohol during treatment. God only knew when I'd be allowed that nectar and ambrosia again.

For two men who own multiple cookbooks and delight in food adventures, we are the most boring and predictable of customers when it comes to pub food. Two pints of Kilkenny Irish Cream Ale, one basket of fries and two baskets of fifteen wings with hot sauce on the side. We've been ordering the same thing for years. The waitress never brings us menus, we just say, "The usual please."

Cognac is frequently the grand finale to such dalliances. But on that night I didn't want to trifle all the time away. I had something serious to discuss with Steve.

Steve and I married sisters. We've been friends from the moment he served all of us a roasted chicken stuffed with bean cassoulet. I knew a good thing when I saw it. That was twenty-odd years ago. We've shared life's laughter and pain ever since.

Steve was aware that Deb couldn't spend five weeks with me in Toronto because of work. She would be there for weeks one and five. Steve had offered to spend week four with me and I gratefully accepted. Both Deb and Steve knew the good, the bad and the ugly of what was coming. Deb and I took an oath to be with each other in sickness and in health, but as the day of reckoning approached, I was wondering what the hell I had gotten Steve into.

I told him that I was worried about putting too much of a strain on our friendship. By the time Steve got to Toronto I'd be in the full throes of radiation side effects. He'd probably end up being a caregiver, quite possibly watching my head regularly hang over a toilet bowl, and not because of excessive cognac consumption. I might want to sleep all the time. I could be in pain. I might be no fun at all.

"Steve, it's a lot to ask of a friend."

He looked me in the eyes and said, "You didn't ask me."

All my trepidation melted away. We clinked glasses and ordered another round.

Tuesday, October 9, 2007, was a great day for Danny Williams, but a demoralizing one for me. It was Election Day and I watched from a distance as Williams was re-elected Premier of Newfoundland and Labrador.

I could have gone back to work after my return from Toronto and played a minor role in our election coverage, but my heart wasn't into it and neither was my head. The impending treatment was occupying all my think-time and frankly, I didn't care about anything else. I would have been a liability at work.

Had I been my normal self, I would have leapt at the chance to be a part of our election special. Four years earlier on Election Day, I was assigned to Premier Roger Grimes' headquarters in Botwood. A disastrous campaign culminated in a disastrous showing at the polls. Twenty minutes after the counting started, the CBC decision desk declared a Progressive Conservative majority government. The Liberals had lost sixteen seats, and power. Danny Williams would be the next premier. This was the worst day of Roger Grimes' political life, but what I remember most was how gracious and poised he was.

He told his disappointed supporters in the hall, "My greatest wish, my greatest wish, is that they absolutely succeed for all of us. Because what we want is a stronger, greater, better Newfoundland and Labrador, and I wish them every single success."

After he came down from the stage I asked him, "Was it Roger Grimes' fault?"

He calmly replied, "I'm sure many people will say that … it was a campaign that I had the responsibility to put together and lead. It was a matter of trying to get a message out and obviously it didn't succeed. The leader must always take full responsibility for that."

That was the Roger Grimes the province saw, composed under great stress. Hours later, after we folded down the satellite dish and were having drinks with his staff back at the Mount Peyton Hotel in nearby Grand Falls, we saw the funny Roger Grimes.

The soon-to-be ex-premier and his wife telephoned from their room. They would like to join us for a drink, but only if no cameras were around. I told his staff, "You can tell the premier the cameras have been put away for the night."

Mary Ann Grimes circled the room before the premier appeared, presumably to make sure that we were true to our word. The premier was upbeat as he walked in. "Who won the pool?" he asked.

I sheepishly put up my hand. NTV's Ken Regular and I correctly predicted the election outcome — 34 Progressive Conservatives, 12 Liberals and 2 New Democrats — and had split the pot of money collected amongst all the reporters.

"Can I buy you a drink, Premier?"

He nodded yes, and I played waiter for him and Mary Ann.

Later, boxes of pizza showed up. The premier had ordered from a pizzeria run by a Greek family. Their pizza was a favourite of his.

Now, there was only a handful of Greeks in Grand Falls in 2003 and only a handful or two more in the rest of province. The premier spent a few minutes chatting with the deliveryman and then excitedly turned to his wife. "Mary Ann, I got the Greek vote!"

The premier could have sulked in his room. He could have licked his wounds in private. But he chose to face adversity with grace and humour. He was a class act.

Being a reporter opens doors that are otherwise closed. Being a cancer patient closes doors that are otherwise open. During Election Day 2007, I heard doors close all around me.

Deb's sister Linda heard milestone news the next day. The Nova Scotia Department of Health had finally approved the drug rituximab for use in hospitals to keep non-Hodgkin's Lymphoma in remission. Linda was absolutely thrilled.

Clinical studies show that two years of maintenance therapy, as the doctors call it, dramatically improves the chances of survival. Maintenance therapy is what some chemo patients have after their chemo treatment stops. Unlike other provinces, Nova Scotia resisted adding rituximab to the list of government paid-for drugs. So Linda started the maintenance therapy at her own expense in a private clinic. The cost was punishing. Plus, it took a toll on Linda's peace of mind. Rituximab was part of her very first chemotherapy cocktail in hospital. She had an allergic reaction and her throat closed over. Even though the nurses got the reaction under control, it scared her. She worried about what would happen if she had another allergic reaction at the private clinic.

Whining is not Linda's style. She adopted the motto: Refuse to give up, refuse to give in! So she wrote letters, made phone calls and generally bugged the hell out of government officials and politicians until they listened to her about the need to include rituximab maintenance therapy in Medicare. She and her doctors had finally won the argument.

Linda so impressed people in the lymphoma community that she was invited to New York to speak at an educational forum on lymphoma. So while I was packing my bags for Toronto, Linda was telling folks in Brooklyn how to right a wrong, and that nobody should have to fight a system when they should be fighting to get well. I was very lucky by comparison. I just had to fight to get well.

The notion of a condemned man's last meal has always intrigued me. What to eat if death were only hours away? Celebrity chef Anthony Bourdain (whom I admire because he scorns fanatical vegetarians, occasionally kills his own food, and has a wickedly funny pen) likes to play The Last Meal Game when he and other masters of the kitchen sit at the end of the bar. Forget your seven-course extravaganza. Bourdain and his colleagues would turn to meatloaf sandwiches and braised ribs for their final sustenance. If they were facing the Grim Reaper, they would pick simple food, not food requiring sixteen hours of frantic fussing in a kitchen where the volume of steam coming out of the chef's ears matches that coming out of the pots. The last meal is no time for hissy fits and temper tantrums. It sounded like good advice.

Only part of me was condemned of course: my taste buds. What tastes did I want to linger forever, just in case I could never savour them again? I craved braised ribs as much as any high-strung chef, but honestly, I've never craved meatloaf sandwiches. I prefer to think of them as a metaphor for comfort food. I decided I wanted a wee bit of elegance added to my comfort food.

I picked lobster. Naturally sweet North Atlantic lobster, boiled in salted water. On the side, melted butter with minced fresh garlic — the perfect dipping sauce. There was coleslaw with a white balsamic vinaigrette, and potato salad with coriander and chipotles. Deb and I washed it all down with a German Riesling. For dessert we had blueberry gratin made with ground almonds and grated lemon peel. Deb had picked the blueberries herself.

I paid attention to flavours like never before. The next morning I was scheduled to fly to Toronto and the damage would start. After that, food would be something to keep me alive, not something to enjoy.

The flight was scheduled to leave at 5:20 am. Deb said Air Canada should advertise it as the get-to-Toronto-in-time-to-see-the-sunrise-flight. My body was just not designed to appreciate pre-dawn travel. I was slumped in a chair by the departure gate. I was sleepy and it wouldn't have taken much to tip me back into a deep slumber. I wondered about the pilot. How do they function at that hour of the morning? I guess someone was pouring coffee into Captain Air Canada because we took off without a hitch.

I watched Bruce Willis save America from a computer megalomaniac. It was just the right diversion for a man embarking on five weeks of radiation treatment. Explosions, car chases and shootings. It was perfectly mindless.

Afterwards, I flipped through brochures from Princess Margaret Hospital. They contained the now familiar and depressing litany of side effects which were coming my way: sunburned appearance, peeling skin, mouth blisters, dry mouth, sore throat, loss of appetite, inability to eat solid food, weight loss, constipation and fatigue. There were practical things I could do to mitigate all of these afflictions, but mostly, I would just have to tough it out. When the radiation stopped, most of the side effects would disappear forever, while others I'd have to learn to live with.

The hospital offered coping with cancer programs. They must have had a prize for the most convoluted name because meditation was called the Mindfulness-Based Stress Reduction Program. That's a name only a psychologist could love. Meanwhile, relaxation training was logically called relaxation training. I could sign up to learn how to manage anxiety through therapeutic touch. Both programs sounded utterly wholesome and dull.

Previously, my mindfulness-based stress reduction involved

Kilkenny ale and cognac. I couldn't do that anymore. I was off the booze until Christmas at the earliest. It made no sense to put a fur ball inside that soon-to-be dry mouth. No, my new approach to managing stress involved diversions on a grand scale. I called it Entertainment Therapy. Number one on the list: tickets to a Bruce Springsteen concert. On the day of my very first radiation treatment I would see the Boss.

I first saw Bruce Springsteen three years earlier in Orlando, Florida. People in the line-up promised that he would make me seventeen again. He did. Few things have thrilled me to the point of making my skin tingle all over. Scoring a goal during the only game I played for my high school hockey team and bringing 500 roaring people to their feet did it. And so did seeing Springsteen. Electricity danced on my skin when he let the last notes of an acoustic version of "Star Spangled Banner" linger in the air as he whipped around the electric guitar hanging on his back and tore into "Born in the USA." I was only thirty feet from him, one foot for every year he took off my life in that instant.

I needed Bruce to create that magic once more. I needed him to make me seventeen again, to bring me back to a time when cancer was something old people had. I needed him to make me cancer-free for a couple of hours.

It was a beautiful sunrise as our taxi drove towards Princess Margaret Hospital Lodge. It was too early to check in, so we piled our luggage into a waiting room and strolled over to Princess Margaret Hospital for my first radiation session.

I was scheduled for 9:25. I scanned my patient card at the front desk. It told the Radiation Therapy Department that I was actually in the waiting room. The computer screen in turn told me that all appointments were on time. I was slotted into treatment unit number 2. Just like the St. John's Cancer Clinic, the radiation machines at Princess Margaret are in basement bunkers. The reception area was bright and welcoming, no hint that it was two floors below ground level. There was a TV on the wall and juice boxes on the coffee table.

A stretcher was wheeled out of one of the rooms. The man on it looked deathly ill. An intravenous bag hung over him and a tube snaked to his arm. I wondered if he was one of the unfortunate souls getting the double whammy of radiation and chemotherapy. I easily could have been him. I made the right call in saying no to chemo. No one should look that sick having something that's supposed to make you better.

"Glenn Deir."

We stood up and walked over to the radiation therapist who called my name. We shook hands as I introduced Deb and myself.

"I'm Lyndon Johnson."

I resisted saying, You're kidding. What luck! A man bearing the same name as a former U.S. president was in charge of my welfare. I took it as an excellent sign. I mean, if a guy named Lyndon Johnson was good enough to sit in the Oval Office, then a guy named Lyndon Johnson was good enough to irradiate my neck.

I couldn't help myself. "Did your mom name you after the president?"

"No, I don't think so."

No matter. From that day, whenever I saw Lyndon, I addressed him as "Mr. President." If it bothered him, he never said a word.

A radiation machine is a bulky, imposing apparatus. It's almost as tall as the room itself, and has a stubby arm that extends out over the bed. At the end of that arm is a horizontal disc that's as wide as a man's shoulders. The arm pivots around the patient, releasing radiation from the disc at different angles.

"Please take off your shirt and lie down."

I noticed that I was already lying on the bed in a manner of speaking. Mr. President and his colleagues had laid out my immobilization mask. We stared at each other for a second.

"What's your birthday?" asked the radiation therapist by the computer. He needed to ensure that they were zapping the right Glenn Deir with the right program.

"January 22, 1958." We would go through this ritual twenty-four more times.

I hopped up on the bed and made myself horizontal. The bed was narrow. My arms wanted to fall off the edge so I tucked my hands under my buttocks. Someone put a wedge-shaped rest underneath the back of my knees. The angle was very comfortable.

There was a great deal of medical gibberish amongst the radiation therapists. A couple of them picked through my chest hair. They were having trouble finding my tattoo. Tattoo is too pretentious sounding, really, to describe the tiny blue dot they were searching for, but it was a permanent mark made the way all tattoos are made — with indelible ink injected under the skin. I had forgotten all about it. The tattoo was put there the day my immobilization mask was cast.

Eventually, someone moved the right chest hair and found the elusive dot. Now they could align the machine properly. Accuracy is paramount when delivering radiation. No sense burning the wrong part of a patient's anatomy. I imagine it's bad for business. They told me that they have just a three-millimetre threshold for error.

"Are you ready?" Mr. President was holding the mask. I nodded. He and the others lowered it over my face, head and shoulders. The snaps along the edge of the mask resembled golf tees. The therapists pushed them into the table. I was pegged and couldn't move without a struggle. They offered to lay a johnny-coat over the exposed part of my chest and stomach. I said no thank you. The room temperature was fine and I didn't want anything else over my skin.

It was time for everyone to leave. When the radiation started they would be safely outside, watching me on a TV monitor. I told the therapists, "Do your best; do your worst." Deb squeezed my hand. She was the last to go.

I didn't feel anything. It was like getting an x-ray. My treatment program released radiation from ten different directions. The disc would hold an angle for a minute at most. The computer program changed the radiation pattern by moving tiny lead bars inside the disc. When it hovered over my face I was able to watch the bars sliding back and forth, forming a new geometric shape every few seconds. It was like a kid's kaleidoscope. I found it perversely cool.

The lead bars made a low rumbling sound, the kind of sound I associate with movie tension tracks when something evil lurking in the bushes is getting ready to strike. I would have to get used to it.

The whole treatment process took about fifteen minutes. The therapists released the snaps and put my ghostly self back on the shelf. I felt fine.

By the time Deb and I got back to the lodge they were ready to check us in. Slight problem though, Deb's suitcase was missing. A nurse soon discovered that another patient had taken it by mistake. The poor man looked so bewildered. Impending cancer treatment must addle the brain.

We were given the room affectionately called the honeymoon suite. It was the only double bed in the lodge. The nurse wryly said, "I think it vibrates." Sadly, she was wrong. The vibrator control didn't work, but both the bed's foot and head could be raised or lowered. That was the extent of lascivious paraphernalia at Princess Margaret Hospital Lodge. No matter, lust was the last thing on my mind. The rest of the day was devoted to Bruce Springsteen.

We linked up with our friends Peter and Debbie from St. John's. Peter is a miracle worker. I don't use that phrase lightly and I don't say it because he's an interventional radiologist who can unblock clogged arteries or stop bleeding deep inside a patient's body. He has brought people back from the edge of death countless times. Yes, he saves lives. All in all, a very handy guy to have around. But as much as I'm in awe of what he does, I could have found half a dozen doctors just like him in any Toronto hospital. No, Peter is a miracle worker because he can routinely score on-the-floor tickets for Bruce Springsteen concerts.

It's a shadowy network. I don't ask many questions. That way I can't get hurt. Some miracle workers can turn water into wine; Peter turned our tickets in the nosebleed section behind the stage into tickets on the floor in front of the stage. And those general admission tickets gave us a chance to stand in The Pit. The Pit is that section of the floor closest to the stage. We might be only feet from Bruce and the E-Street Band. Now that's a miracle.

We dutifully lined up outside the Air Canada Centre, along with hundreds of other fans holding general admission tickets. Our merry band had grown to six. Another radiologist from St. John's and her boyfriend joined us. I was starting to feel like a Saudi Arabian sheik. I had two doctors in tow. Could anyone else in the line-up say that?

Bruce's security team gave a numbered, happy-face wristband to everyone in the line-up. I was number 90. At 5:15 the head of Bruce's security wandered by with the lottery jar. Gerry (How does Peter know these things?) stopped by a little blond girl just behind me. She was ten or eleven. She would get the honour of picking the winning number. The person holding that number and about 400 others behind him or her would be in The Pit.

As her hand was reaching into the jar, I was thinking, Sweet little girl, angelic little girl, pick number 90. She carefully chose one ticket, just as she had been instructed. She pulled it out and read, "80."

"We're in The Pit!" I shouted. There were hugs, high-fives and cheering. The celebration rolled down the line.

"Wait!" said Gerry. "It's a mistake. It's actually 380." Our section of the line fell into a stony silence. Hugs, high-fives and cheering erupted well behind us.

I glared at the little girl and thought, You are the Devil's spawn.

We would have to be satisfied with the consolation prize of standing farther back on the floor, somewhere beyond the blue line if you were judging distance by sections of a hockey rink.

We kidded that it might be time to go to plan B: play the cancer card. Put me in a wheelchair, have my personal physicians speak to Gerry and explain that the Adult Wish Foundation had promised to let me see Bruce up close. Would God really hold it against me on Judgment Day that I stretched the truth to get within an arm's reach of Bruce Springsteen? Tempting, but it was only flirtatious humour.

Peter has never been my doctor; we've only ever been friends. His one bit of medical advice when he heard about my impending radiation treatment was, "Just make sure you're going through this for the right reason." I guess the breast cancer testing fiasco back home was on his mind too.

The tally of specialists who had touched my cancer was larger than most people get: three pathologists, two radiation oncologists, two ear nose and throat surgeons, and a medical oncologist. I had gotten a second opinion and then some. There was no doubt about what needed to be done.

The security team began handing out the coveted second wristband to the chosen ones. And then another miracle. They went from number 380 to the end of the line and still had wristbands left over. So they started with number 1 and kept coming. The cut-off was 110. We were headed to The Pit after all.

Sweet little girl, angelic little girl, I thought.

When the doors opened around seven we scampered inside. Two wristbands, no stopping. We took a wrong turn and got lost briefly in a corridor full of doors leading to corporate boxes. Oops. We beat a hasty retreat and were soon staking out our territory in The Pit. Maybe the Adult Wish Foundation really did exist. We were closer to the stage than in Orlando. Bruce would be just fifteen feet away.

The lights went down and I wasn't glowing in the dark, if that's what you're wondering. But my spirits were glowing.

The crowd called, "Bruuuuuuuuuce!" A carnival organ rose out of the stage. The circus sounds seemed appropriate enough considering his new album was called *Magic*.

Bruce yelled from the blackness, "Is there anybody alive out there?" The crowd roared back and Bruce launched into his new single "Radio Nowhere." Sparks jumped all over my body. Steve Van Zandt in his trademark bandana, Clarence Clemons with his trademark saxophone, the Boss strutting around the stage, all of them almost close enough to touch. They were playing every song just for me. Cancer wasn't all bad. It had dropped me in the lap of Bruce Springsteen and the E-Street Band.

The show was Springsteen anthem after Springsteen anthem. My favourite was "Badlands." I'd chosen it as my theme song for the next five weeks.

Badlands, you gotta live it everyday
Let the broken hearts stand
As the price you've gotta pay
We'll keep pushing 'till it's understood
And these Badlands start treating us good.

The lights went up. The crowd was on its feet. My eyes left the stage and I slowly twisted on the spot, scanning the thousands of dancing fans around me. Even the folks in the highest seats at the back of the Air Canada Centre were thrilled to the core. These Badlands were indeed treating us good. It was a moment of bliss. I was seventeen again and I was cancer-free.

Two hours and twenty minutes of Entertainment Therapy zapped away all the worry. The afterglow lasted through the night. I dreamt that a nurse came into my room and saw my blotchy beard.

"Don't worry," she said, "I'll fix that with a beard pill."

Holiday Lover

I was astonished at how quickly my radiation treatment felt like a normal part of my daily routine. By day three it was familiar: a necessary chore like brushing my teeth. Nothing more outstanding than that. All my appointments were scheduled for early morning, so Deb and I were free to play tourist for much of the day, which suited me just fine because I am a Holiday Lover by nature.

Being labelled a Holiday Lover is harmless in Canada, but if you're declared a Holiday Lover in Japan, your career is in tatters. You won't even be considered for middle management positions, much less the big bucho (boss). My Wednesday night beer-drinking companion told me the story. John and I were regulars at the Hiki Bar in Shibuya district, just a five-minute walk from NHK. Hanlon-san, as the Japanese called him, was the dean of the CBC alumni at Nippon Hoso Kyokai (Japan Broadcasting Corporation) and we became fast friends. Our Wednesday night gabfests were full of shoptalk, CBC memories, tall tales, office politics and pontificating on the mysteries of Japanese culture.

John told me about a Japanese colleague who approached him one night after scouring the newsroom. He was looking for someone and wondered if John had seen him. John replied that he had earlier in the evening.

"You know Hanlon-san," the colleague said with a look of complete disgust, "he is a Holiday Lover."

That was the most contemptuous thing he could attach to a Japanese salaryman. Never mind that the poor fellow had probably worked well in excess of his regular eight-hour shift. The word was out. He would not bleed for the company and therefore this man was deemed a labour-shirking cur. Others on his team had work to do and he was not there to help, or at least offer moral support. Scandalous! He was indeed a Holiday Lover.

Hanlon-san teased me about being a Holiday Lover too. Not undeservedly, I might add. While living in Tokyo I took vacations to Italy, St. John's, Kyoto, Sapporo, Hawaii, Australia, South Korea and New Zealand. Hanlon-san knew a Holiday Lover when he saw one.

It was true. My days of bleeding for the company were over. I was no longer willing to routinely punch in ten-hour shifts, sacrifice days off, eat sandwiches instead of a cooked dinner, and generally let work consume my life. Fortunately, NHK didn't expect that. As a gaijin (foreigner), I got a pass from the demands imposed on a Japanese salaryman.

However, if one is going to take the emperor's yen, then one has to give the emperor a good day's work. I greatly admired that characteristic and wished people in the west could be a little more Japanese sometimes. NHK staff put their shoulders to the wheel immediately when work needed to be done. There was no saying, "I'll be there in a minute." Conversations stopped in mid-sentence to assist a colleague or to answer the boss. When I heard the call, "Glenn-san!" my reply had to be a quick "Hai!" *Yes, I'm coming.*

Being a gaijin and a Holiday Lover, I was free to book two-week vacations. None of my Japanese colleagues ever did that. One week was as much as they dare ask for. They might spend two days travelling to and from Hawaii just to get five days on Waikiki beach. I once asked Susumu why he never requested more time off. "Oh, I couldn't," he replied, "then other people in the office would have to do my work." What devotion. I hope he doesn't work himself to death. It happens in Japan with frightening regularity. The Japanese even have a word for it — karoshi — death from overwork.

I've always wondered if Sasaki-san died from karoshi. One Monday I was greeted with the news that something awful had happened over the weekend. Sasaki-san had dropped dead. Speculation around the office was that he died from a heart attack. He was one of the few overweight Japanese I'd seen. Dead at forty-six, leaving to mourn a wife and two kids.

Sasaki-san was responsible for the feature stories that we ran in the back half of the program. They were wonderfully eclectic reports, ranging from clearing landmines in Cambodia to saving tigers in Russia. They were prepared by NHK's foreign correspondents and Sasaki-san's job was to turn the Japanese version into an English version. We worked together daily. He was always polite and easy going.

In Japan, friends and colleagues of the deceased help pay for the funeral. The family is given a cash gift. There is a sliding scale, depending on one's relationship with the deceased. Okawa-san recommended I give 5000 yen, or about 55 dollars. Hideshi, one of our hosts, went to the store with me to make sure I bought the appropriate card. We all saw the potential peril of my coming back with a card that read, "Congratulations on your retirement." There was nothing discreet about how much each of us contributed. The yen amount was marked on the front of the envelope, while my name and address were on the back.

The right dress was critical. I had to wear black. Period. I had a black jacket, but it was matched with olive pants. The office voted that down. The dark navy suit was considered the best option. No one would take offence. A white shirt and black tie were also mandatory. Problem number 2: I didn't have a black tie. Not to worry, Hideshi assured me, they sold them at subway kiosks for just such occasions. Apparently, Japan is full of men who need black ties on short notice.

I arrived at the funeral home sporting a new black tie, purchased only minutes before in the subway station. I was in the overflow room along with dozens of other people. There were several eulogies. I heard the phrase NHK many times, no doubt telling everyone what a loyal employee he was and how the NHK family would miss him.

The only odd thing about the experience was the music piped in during the ceremony. It was very melodramatic and at times bordered on being silly. I half expected a chase scene to break out at any moment. I was told later that it was Sasaki-san's favourite piece.

The emotion was real and familiar. There was plenty of sobbing in our room. He had good friends and they were heartbroken. We were invited into the main room to say a formal goodbye. The front was full of flowers and in the middle was a painting of Sasaki-san. We marched in threes toward the altar and bowed to the family. I had been well coached. Keep my hands by my side and bend at the hip about 45 degrees. His wife and children bowed back. We each took a little incense and sprinkled it on a stick of burning charcoal.

Sasaki-san's casket seemed to be made out of particleboard, perhaps because he was going to be cremated. It had a window over his face. A chance for one last look, I thought. After a second bow to the family we slipped back into the overflow room. It was our turn now to receive a gift. The family must show gratitude for your presence and condolence money. Everyone was given a box of tea and a handkerchief.

The funeral home staff lifted the cover off Sasaki-san's casket and we were invited to lay flowers on his body. By the end, it looked as though he were lying in a flowerbed, completely covered except for his face. It was colourful, peaceful and dignified.

His wife spoke for a few minutes, thanking everyone for coming and explaining what a shock it was. Unfortunately, his children had found him. The boy was about fourteen, the girl eleven. So young to witness something so awful. They called the fire department and the paramedics tried to save him, but it was too late.

No, Glenn-san will not die from overwork. No one will write karoshi as the official cause of death on my death certificate. They will not find me slumped over a desk with a half-written story on my computer. My time on the radiation table only steeled my resolve to be a Holiday Lover

Dr. Waldron said a cheery hello. This was the first of my weekly check-ups during radiation treatment. I had no symptoms to report and I felt great. Four sessions down, twenty-one more to go.

The last thing a busy radiation oncologist needs is another form to fill out, but that's exactly what I needed from Dr. Waldron. The Case Manager with CBC's Health and Wellness Office wanted a medical absence report completed.

I had already sent a letter from Dr. Norman in St. John's. It stated that I was off work in early September for "two surgical procedures" and I would need an additional "three months leave for further therapy." I was pleased that it was vague. I felt CBC had every right to determine if I was a malingerer, whether I was feigning illness, but the prospect of revealing more rankled me. It was none of their business. Dr. Norman's letter had disclosed enough as it was. She identified herself as a radiation oncologist at the Cancer Care Program with Eastern Health. You didn't need to be a rocket scientist to figure out what was happening to me.

Still, it wasn't sufficient. An official CBC form was required. The Case Manager assured me that the information would be kept confidential and wouldn't be shared with anyone outside her office. She sounded sincere, but I doubted that my medical condition would stay secret for long. Secrets always have a way of squirting out at the CBC. We're terrible gossips, and nosy journalists to boot.

Dr. Waldron had no choice but to answer the CBC's questions truthfully. Under nature of the illness he wrote carcinoma oropharynx (throat cancer). Is the patient under active treatment? Yes, radiation treatments for five weeks. Has the patient undergone surgery? Yes, neck and tonsil biopsy. Nature of restrictions? Cannot work at all. Expected date of return? March 1, 2008.

Well, not much left to the imagination there. The Case Manager was about to be as well informed as my wife.

Dr. Waldron gave me a couple of prescriptions. "You'll be needing these." The first was for liquid codeine. I sighed. Codeine would be both my angel of mercy and tormenting demon. Codeine is a member of the opioid family, a particularly addictive clan that includes morphine, opium and heroin. But if used as directed, I shouldn't become addicted to liquid codeine. It would control my pain. Mr. President and his cabinet were burning my throat, and pain would inevitably come.

If only codeine were side-effect free. It's not. Constipation is a common consequence. I was on codeine for a week when my left tonsil was removed. I was also taking a stool softener and laxative to counteract the codeine's binding qualities. Despite the medicinal assistance, having a bowel movement was like passing rocks. There was plenty of squeezing my lower abdomen muscles and bearing down. I imagined the drugs as soldiers in trench warfare. Every so often a platoon sergeant would lead a charge over the top to reclaim no man's land. Neither side could score outright victory. It was a stalemate. There was no hope of peaceful passage until the two sides stopped shelling each other and went home.

The second prescription was for a mucositis mouthwash. The medication info sheet made it sound like wine. I was promised an orange-red suspension with a fruity scent. All right then, I'll take a case.

I was less enthusiastic after reading the fine print. Mucositis is a medical term for mouth sores. The mouthwash would reduce pain and prevent yeast infections. It was one-third lidocaine, an anaesthetic for temporarily numbing my mouth; one-third nystatin, an antifungal drug; and one-third unsweetened cherry Kool-Aid. The Kool-Aid was there simply for flavouring. The concoction's chief function was to help me get food down by deadening my mouth and throat.

I was determined to drink neither prescription until I absolutely needed it. I asked Dr. Waldron when I should start using my dental trays and fluoride gel. Right away, he said. Great. My bedtime ritual would now include coating my teeth in goop before kissing Deb goodnight.

I never imagined that I would hear my mother's voice again, but I did at the end of the week. Deb and I rented a car and drove to Hamilton to spend the weekend with my cousin Ann and her husband Kurt. Ann had stumbled across a treasure trove while sorting through her father's belongings. Stuffed away in a closet were letters from my mother to her brother Clive (Ann's dad) and sister Vivian, some written before I was born and some after. I was about to get a glimpse into my mother's life half a century ago.

Mom had been dead thirty-two years, but as soon as I saw that crisp writing I recognized it instantly. What penmanship they practiced in those days. My own handwriting is a scrawl by comparison. Mom's words were so legible. I offered to read the letters aloud. We sat around the living room and as I lifted the words off the paper, I could hear Mom speaking them in my mind.

Jan. 9th/56
My Dear Viv,
Here I am at last to try and bring you up to date on the fast moving events of the last month. Many things will be forgotten I'm sure, but I'm sure you'll forgive me if I slip up in places. If you don't want to part with this letter maybe you could type a copy for Clive, as I can't write the whole lot too many times.
On Sunday morning at 9 a.m. Dec. 11th I received a long distance call from Dad asking me to come on the train. Of course I said yes if needed. So he proceeded to say mother was ill, seriously ill and lastly critical. The way he said critical I judged the worse and asked him outright, so he said yes. The shock I got cannot be described. If the tables had been reversed

it wouldn't have been because I've lived with that for years. We got in touch with Lloyd [Mom's brother] at Gander and broke the news to him. It was an awful day here. I got to the station that night in a jeep. Nothing else moving. I set off at midnight. Arrived Clarenville 7 a.m. where Lloyd met me. A car was going through to Bonavista following the plough, so we took off and reached Bonavista at 12.30 with no worse a mishap, except having to make the second run for Summerville hill. I have so much to be thankful for that it helps me over the dark spots. Dad is a broken old man in many ways, but he rallied after we got there and bore up very bravely ...

Mother looked very peaceful and was laid out in her brown dress. The casket was brown, lined with cream satin. I can't begin to tell you how kind people were. It would fill a book. We received over 300 telegrams, cards, letters etc., and 26 wreaths. Parcels of food galore and visitors too numerous to mention. The service at the home was beautiful. The U.C. [United Church] and C of E [Church of England] ministers held a joint service both there and at the grave. The hymns at the house were "The Lord's My Shepherd" and "Lead Kindly Light", at the grave "Abide With Me". It was a fairly good day, but a few flurries of snow fell. We got through it all as good as can be expected, and I got the fires going and the blinds up and lights on by the time they got back from the service ...

Lou can tell you how Mother knew she was going and told her so. However, that Saturday she never was as well for a long time or ate so well. Dad came home at 9.30 p.m. tired and wanted to go to bed, but she had so much to do before she could go, he undressed and lay on the daybed. At 12.30 she called him saying she was ready to go to bed and said, "I feel a bit sick" — then before he could get off the couch she fell to the floor. When he picked her up her left side was all gone. He got her on the couch and the pulse wasn't too bad, but in half an hour she just sank deeper and deeper into a coma and by 3.30 was gone. She vomited a lot and he couldn't leave her to go for help in case she'd choke. So he was with her alone when she went, and in fact had her just about laid out when help finally arrived ...

Don't mourn for Mother she's at peace, our biggest worry is with the living. Now don't think Dad was hard to handle, he wasn't. But you know how wrapped up he is in medicine and he just can't tear himself away from Bonavista ... I weep inwardly and ask for guidance. I can only pray all will be well and eventually things will all work together for good.

He phoned me Friday and keeps telling me not to worry, but I can't help it. He cries a lot now especially when he said goodbye to me, and you know that's not like him. I can't bear to think of him there alone. I don't think he'll starve — the neighbours are too kind — but you know he can't cook for brewis, or wash, or keep a house ...

Forgot to say Mother's death was attributed to a cerebral haemorrhage ... Feel very tired now Viv and 6 a.m. comes very soon, so guess I'll say good night and hope I haven't left you more confused than ever with my ramblings. Do write me again very soon.
Love from all of us,
Kay

I had never heard the story before. My grandmother died in my grandfather's arms. He wasn't just Chesley Alexander Forbes, he was Dr. Chesley Alexander Forbes. Over forty years of practicing medicine and he still couldn't save her. I never knew him or her, but I felt sorry for them both and for my mother. I knew the pain of burying parents, but after reading my mother's letter it was so easy to see how no generation has a monopoly on grief. It's all been felt before.

My mother was right to worry about my grandfather. He died two days after she wrote the letter to Aunt Viv. Mom brought stoicism to everything in her life, including battles with cancer, first in her breast and later in her brain. She faced life's crises with dignity and a sensible perseverance. All these years after she was gone and she was still leading by example, no doubt expecting me to follow.

My mother's letters also reminded me how lucky I am to be alive during the age of universal health care. My dad wasn't well when I was born. The financial strain showed itself in Mom's letters.

Jack will be off pay from now on, till he goes back. It could be much worse so I'm not grumbling. It's hard to make the kids understand though. They think I'm John D. Rockefeller.

A year later.

Jack goes back for another check-up as soon as the reply comes. Hope he'll be clear of pills etc., as he is a human drug store. The doctor's bills I'm sure will be flooring, of course that's all we've seen this year.

That Medicare card in my wallet is my Gold card. I shudder to think what the bill might be for two surgeries, CT and MRI scans, pathology reports, consultations with several specialists and five weeks of radiotherapy. I'd probably have to sell my house to pay for it. Mom and Dad lived in a time when people actually did that; an illness could bankrupt a family. I had no bills whatsoever. Thank you, thank you, thank you, Tommy Douglas. Canada's father of Medicare truly deserved to be voted the Greatest Canadian of them all.

The letters were a wonderful snapshot of my parents' life circa 1958. My sister Judy was a self-absorbed teenager who exasperated my mother. My sister Barb was on the verge of marrying an American serviceman, and Mom was anxious about her getting pregnant right away. Ann also made appearances in the letters.

Kiss Ann for us.

That made my cousin sit up. A subsequent letter had even more affection and there was talk of a new baby, but not a girl.

How are you Evelyn? Do hope by now you are in and out of hospital and that your new addition is a son with both of you in tip-top shape ... How is dear little Ann? ... XXXXX for Ann.

Ann was beaming. Her Aunt Kay was giving her all the ammunition she needed for the next clash of the Forbes sisters. It just kept getting worse for Lynn.

How glad I was to hear Evelyn, you were safely over it, and although probably a bit disappointed over the outcome, still happy to hear that your second little girl arrived in perfect condition.

Ann couldn't wait any longer. She dialled Lynn's number in Orillia. Little sister needed to be told immediately that she was supposed to be a boy, and that her gender was a source of great sorrow to the entire Forbes clan. Oh, the indignity. Ann said she obviously had to be the favourite niece because of all the nice things my mother said about her. They were laughing, thank God. The last thing I needed was a sibling rivalry induced screaming match.

Seeing my infant self through my mother's eyes was at first sweet, but then embarrassing.

Glenn is growing like a top, but seems backward to me as he makes no effort to sit up.

Backward! My mother said I was backward. I have a university degree, I work as a television journalist with the finest news organization in Canada, and I'm writing a bloody book, but all my mother saw was a seven-month-old baby who was too stunned to sit up. Ann and Deb were hooting. Apparently, no man is a god to his mother either.

Saturday night saw all of us at a fundraising dance for Ann's dragon boat team. It was a great diversion. The band did a terrific
cover of Carrie Underwood's "Before He Cheats." The lead singer
said, "It's my new favourite song." If I were her husband, I'd be
taking extra care not to piss her off because she looked perfectly
capable of swinging a Louisville Slugger.

The highlight of the evening was Meatloaf's "Paradise by the
Dashboard Light." Another anthem from my teens to bookend
the week. Deb and I were dancing. I felt so good that I got cocky
and committed the one act I should not have — hubris. The
ancient Greeks warned against it and so did Con several months
earlier. I ignored their advice and let arrogant confidence swell
up. Well, I thought, if this is the worst radiation can do to me,
bring it on.

The next day I drove Deb to the Toronto airport. She had to return to work in St. John's. We hugged briefly at the curb and she
was gone. I drove into the city and returned the rented car. As I
crossed Yonge Street on my walk back to the lodge I realized I
was hungry. What luck; there was a sushi restaurant.

I'm sure I ate my body weight in raw fish while living in
Tokyo. My favourite sushi memory comes from a night when
Susumu, Murakami-san and Naoto invited me to tag along for
an after-work nosh. We strolled from NHK to a kaiten sushi
restaurant. Kaiten is Japanese for revolve, and inside, small plates
of sushi were parading in front of the diners on a conveyor belt
that went round and round. When you see something you like
you simply pick it off the belt. Your bill is calculated by adding
up the number of plates piled in front of you.

Japanese waitresses are usually demure, so I was startled
when the hostess held up her hand to stop us. She pointed at a
sign on the wall and said something sternly to Susumu.

He was laughing as he translated. "She says, 'Are you sure that you can eat at least seven plates? You must eat seven plates.'" We all agreed that we were starving and seven plates wouldn't be a problem.

We had barely sat down when the chefs behind the counter started yelling, "Don't be shy. Shout out if you want something." Not only were we being strong-armed to gorge ourselves, we had to eat quickly. Tiny signs on the conveyor belt implored us to finish eating within thirty minutes.

There was no such pressure at the Toronto sushi restaurant. I ordered salmon and tuna rolls, my favourites. They should have been delicious, but something was wrong. The sushi didn't taste right; the flavours were strange and not at all enjoyable.

The Greek gods had heard my foolish challenge to bring on the radiation, and now I was paying for my vanity. Idiot!

Radiation Man

Week two of radiation pretty well wiped the smirk off my face. Radiation has a cumulative effect; the treatments pile on top of each other. By mid-week I was talking as if I had just returned from the dentist with my mouth full of Novocain.

Mr. President predicted it would happen by the following Monday. *It* was a sore throat. By then, he expected I'd be changing my diet to soft foods. So far, I had been able to eat everything, though I was enjoying nothing. My taste buds had turned against me and all food had a metallic taste. Lyndon Johnson could have been wrong, but not likely. He had seen hundreds of radiation patients like me and he could probably pinpoint changes to the exact hour. I would have been a fool to bet against him.

No, in all his years of irradiating people he had never seen anyone avoid side effects. It was simply a matter of degree: How red would I get? How sore would I be? The President's word was law. However, he offered one glimmer of hope amongst that glum news. "You might get super powers."

Now, there was an enticing side effect. I didn't scoff at the suggestion, I embraced it. After all, a radioactive spider turned Peter Parker into Spiderman. I could call myself Radiation Man. I already had the mask; I only needed the rest of the costume. Mr. President was a little vague about what super powers I might acquire, but one day there might be a comic named after me and my ghostly face would be plastered on kids' pyjamas. The Amazing Radiation Man. Sugoi, as the Japanese might say. *Wow!*

Bring it on, I thought, and this time I felt full of excited anticipation, not arrogance.

The radiation therapists were always friendly and politely asked how I was doing. They tried to make it personal, but in reality, it was an assembly line. They pushed twenty-eight people through a day in my unit alone. In one way, all twenty-eight of us were in the room at the same time. All our immobilization masks were neatly stacked on shelves. Twenty-eight heads, no torsos. They'd grab the appropriate one as a new patient wandered in.

The Evil Glenn thought of these people as torturers. Every day they got their hands on me, I got sicker. I wanted to say after a session, "That was great! Do you think I could try the thumbscrews tomorrow?" Oh, but no, I dutifully thanked them and cheerily said, "Have a good day. See you later."

Prisoners in the Tower of London would sometimes offer the executioner a valuable piece of jewellery just before getting their heads lopped off to ensure that he did a good job. Maybe that was my problem. I wasn't offering bribes to the radiation therapists. Perhaps if I had, they would have turned up the dial and I could have gotten the awful mess over with in one fell swoop.

My friends kept my email account full of uplifting notes. One came from Marc in Tokyo. He wrote, "Ganbatte kudasai." Ganbatte is ubiquitous in Japan and is a very useful word. It can mean go for it, don't give up, carry on, hang in there or keep going. And because Marc has adopted the manners of a polite Japanese, he added please to his encouragement.

I always thought that the unofficial office motto at NHK had to be "Ganbatte!"

The word certainly crossed my mind during a meeting in

the middle of the newsroom to outline upcoming changes in our show. It was quite unremarkable until a young woman keeled over in front of Okawa-san. She toppled from her chair and landed at his feet. Everyone scrambled to get her to the couch in the middle of the meeting area. Someone kindly laid a coat over her and she curled into a fetal position.

After the flash of excitement, the most extraordinary thing happened — the meeting carried on. The woman didn't stir. In that fine Japanese tradition of not complaining, she endured a lecture on television news production surrounded by twenty or so journalists without so much as a whimper. Ganbatte!

The meeting didn't stop again until two people in white jackets showed up — the NHK first-aid team. Moments later, six men in blue smocks and white helmets rushed in. They were paramedics from the Tokyo Fire Department and they were carrying bags of equipment, including a defibrillator. They seemed disappointed to learn that they wouldn't be jump-starting anyone's heart. After checking the woman's pulse and other vital signs, the paramedics strapped her into a chair/stretcher contraption and wheeled her out. With the distractions gone, it was back to the meeting.

A Japanese needed a healthy dose of ganbatte to navigate the complicated world of Japanese hierarchy. I got glimpses from time to time. One night after the show, the Chief News Editor asked my opinion about our coverage of President George W. Bush's trip to New Delhi. India and the U.S. had just signed a nuclear cooperation agreement and our coverage concentrated on the trade implications of the president's visit. I told Sakane-san that I thought we should have examined how Pakistan viewed this nuclear deal, since it occasionally goes to war with India. Or consider North Korea's position, since the U.S. was demanding that the North abandon its nuclear programs because the Americans wanted to reduce the nuclear threat in the region.

"That's what I wanted to do," said Sakane-san, "but *he* insisted on the economic story." Sakane-san was pointing his finger at Ikeda-san.

"But you're the boss," I said in a puzzled voice.

"Yes, but he is older, and I had to do it."

Age trumped authority in the NHK newsroom. Japanese harmony is based on accepting decisions you don't agree with and knowing your boundaries. After that episode, I sometimes saw resentment smouldering behind the smiles and bows of our workplace etiquette. Ganbatte!

Okawa-san needed the occasional "Ganbatte!" as well. Over lunch he once told me that the day hadn't been good. He had just received his annual bonus and it had been drastically cut. This was on top of having his salary reduced by 20 per cent the previous spring, when he turned fifty-seven. That was policy at NHK and perfectly legal. The corporate culture decreed that at age fifty-seven an employee was past his prime and it was time to move on. The wage rollback was a push to get an employee out the door by age sixty. I was mortified and offered to buy lunch. "Yes," said Okawa-san, "that was my plan all along." I loved his dry humour.

Looking back on it, it's a wonder Okawa-san let me anywhere near Japan. When I heard he would fly all the way to St. John's to interview me, I excitedly told my friend Bryan.

"Don't mention the war," said Bryan.

We both exploded in laughter. That classic sketch from the British sitcom *Fawlty Towers*, when rude hotelier Basil Fawlty goose-steps his way through the dining room to the disgust of his German guests, always left Bryan and me in convulsions. We watched it countless times and regularly incorporated Basil's "Don't mention the war" into our banter.

I studied Japanese business etiquette in preparation for Okawa-san's arrival. Turn the writing on my business card towards him, hold it in two hands, make sure my card was beneath his during the exchange, remark on his card, leave it on the table during the interview and never, ever write on it.

"NHK will not make you a star," said Okawa-san. He wanted me to understand that I would be a re-writer and not a foreign correspondent. His questions were the most wide-ranging and personal of any interview I've ever been subjected to. "How is your health?" "How much money do you earn?" "Are you a hunter?"

"Well, yes actually, I do hunt — caribou."

Okawa-san perked up. I told him about my expeditions into the Newfoundland interior. He seemed genuinely interested. I didn't know whether this was his way of weeding out the psychopaths or finding a truly unique specimen to bring back to the NHK World newsroom.

We finished the interview around lunch hour. Okawa-san presented me with a beautifully wrapped box. "It is a key case." I was embarrassed. I had nothing for him. There was a lapse in my research. I had been told about the importance of looking after guests in Japanese culture, so I decided to offer my services as a tour guide after work.

"Okawa-san, I don't want to breach any protocols, but if you would like —"

Okawa-san jumped in. "To have lunch, yes."

I had to scramble. Deb had the car at home and I needed it now. It seemed to take forever for her to arrive.

"Perhaps she is putting on makeup," said Okawa-san.

The fact that Deb dropped everything to attend to the needs of her husband's business affairs likely impressed Okawa-san. Japanese wives are expected to do such things without question, and NHK had never hired a married foreigner for this job. Okawa-san had asked a lot of questions about Debbie-san, perhaps trying to determine if she would interfere with Glenn-san's commitment to NHK. After the introductions, Deb made a quick exit. She did all the right things.

Okawa-san and I strolled out to the car. "It is Korean," observed Okawa-san. Oops. I was driving a Hyundai Elantra. Korea and Japan are rivals in manufacturing; selling cars overseas is a matter of great pride for both nations. Theirs is a complicated relationship. Both rose out of the ashes of mid-twentieth century wars to become economic giants in Asia, but Korea has never fully forgiven Japan for annexing the Korean Peninsula in 1910. Japan ruled Korea for thirty-five years.

Don't mention the war. Basil's words were bouncing around my head. "I used to drive a Nissan Sentra," I sputtered, "but when I needed a new car, the Hyundai was so much cheaper."

Okawa-san nodded. The nod said, "I understand" not "I approve."

After lunch, I drove Okawa-san around downtown St. John's. What luck! There was a Japanese fishing boat tied up on the waterfront, flying the sun flag. On and on I went about how the Japanese love Newfoundland capelin, how the capelin roll in on our beaches to spawn, and how Newfoundlanders have dried and salted capelin for centuries. I was a fountain of knowledge until it occurred to me that Okawa-san probably didn't have a clue what fish I was talking about. Capelin is an English word. He knew the fish by another name and I had no idea what capelin was in Japanese. Explaining that it's a small fish eaten by others wouldn't really explain very much at all.

"Let's go up Signal Hill," I said, hoping to shift attention away from my linguistic shortcomings. It was a beautiful afternoon and Signal Hill offers a million dollar view of St. John's. I prattled on about Marconi receiving the first wireless transatlantic radio signal on Signal Hill.

"NHK started here." Okawa-san laughed.

We wandered over to the part of the hill that overlooks the mouth of the harbour — The Narrows.

"What is that over there?" asked Okawa-san. He was pointing down to Fort Amherst. I knew he wasn't referring to the lighthouse. No doubt his question had to do with the remains of the gun batteries that were built during World War II.

I was trapped. "They had big guns there during the war. They also had a net stretched across the channel to keep submarines out of the harbour. GERMAN submarines."

Okawa-san nodded. The nod said, "I understand" not "I approve."

I wondered, How will I ever live this down? Bryan will crucify me.

My only hope lay in Basil's faulty logic. "I mentioned the war once, but I think I got away with it all right."

Okawa-san and I walked around for a few more minutes. "You will not see green like this in Tokyo, only concrete. I will go back to the hotel now."

A month later, I received the nicest rejection letter ever to pass through the mail slot in my front door. NHK managers were very impressed with my impromptu tour around the city, but the position had gone to someone else. That'll teach me to mention the war. I found out later that the successful candidate was Lorne Saxsberg. Lorne was a star announcer on CBC Newsworld. He had golden pipes for vocal chords and they had dazzled NHK World. I lost fair and square.

A year later, NHK wanted to borrow another journalist from the CBC and I applied again, with Okawa-san's encouragement. Once more he flew to St. John's. I picked him up at the airport and this time there was no formal interview, we just went straight to lunch. We chatted over blackened cod, everything from the NHK job to life in Tokyo. We concluded with an exchange of gifts. He gave me an NHK mouse pad and I gave him a CBC mug.

"I haven't had much time for shopping," said Okawa-san. He needed to buy omiyage. Omiyage is more than a souvenir. It's a present of food for the office to make amends for abandoning your colleagues. They've stayed behind working diligently, while you're off somewhere having a good time. I suggested jams made from Newfoundland berries. We wandered over to Auntie Crae's for some taste testing. His staff got mini-bottles of bakeapple jam, while Mrs. Okawa got a bottle of partridgeberry jam.

Okawa-san had a big smile on his face as we shook hands at the airport. "Good things can happen while you sleep." A month later, a letter offering me the position of Broadcast Specialist landed in the same spot as the rejection letter the year before.

"I GOT THE JOB. I'M GOING TO TOKYO." There was no one in the house to come running, but yelling seemed like the logical thing to do. I read the letter over and over to make sure I wasn't hallucinating. The words didn't change. I instantly had a thousand things to do and only one thing not to do. "Don't mention the war," I said to myself.

I was walking along College Street on my way to a radiation appointment when I was reminded of what an obscure cancer I had. I stopped by a Canadian Cancer Society poster. *We Fight All Cancers*, it proudly said. The poster listed off the famous six: leukemia, colorectal, lung, breast, cervical and prostate. I smiled to myself and speculated that the poster would have to stretch halfway around the block before it would mention tonsil cancer. I don't think there will ever be a Run for the Cure that focuses on tonsil cancer. Maybe an Eat Ice Cream for the Cure event. The cancer survivors and their families could hold it in a phone booth.

"Don't laugh," I said to Dr. Waldron. "I'd like to ask you about acupuncture and how that might affect saliva production."

He didn't laugh. While Deb's sister Linda was in New York she met a doctor who thinks that acupuncture could possibly alleviate dry mouth. The doctor said tests in Sweden showed that acupuncture needles increased blood flow to the salivary glands and might even stimulate tissue regeneration.

"I'm not familiar with the study. I think there can be a role for traditional medicine, but I don't want you doing anything to cause more inflammation in your neck while we're treating you."

He had a point. They were doing enough damage, thank you very much. Dr. Waldron suggested that I wait until after I healed, before trying acupuncture. I told him I would, but he went on. I must have touched a nerve.

"One in three Canadians will get cancer, and of that group, 30 per cent will die from it. I've had patients literally sell the family farm, with the family's approval, trying to buy a miracle cure in Mexico. Do people really think if there was a cure out there that multi-national companies wouldn't go after it? They'd buy it up and make millions selling it."

There was no need for me to sell the family farm. They were talking cure for me, a 90 per cent chance. How desperate some people must be when the word cure is no longer part of their conversations with doctors. I wondered how I'd react if Dr. Waldron were saying, "I'm sorry, there's nothing more I can do. You should go home and get your affairs in order." I might be tempted to sell the family farm too.

If you judge a man by the company he keeps, then I was guilty of being among the wicked. The honeymoon suite at Princess Margaret Hospital Lodge and I had parted company. Once Deb went home, I was moved into a room with two single beds and acquired a roommate. I was impressed when I heard that he was a cartoonist, and then thrilled to discover that he had sold cartoons to *Playboy* and *Hustler* magazines. Every prurient instinct I had made my ears stand up. Tales about porn king Larry Flynt were far more entertaining than swapping cancer details.

I was a bit of a lone wolf at the lodge. I tended not to mix much, largely because I wanted to avoid the "What are you in for?" conversations. Despite my best efforts though, I was occasionally roped into such chats, usually over lunch in the cafeteria. I was still the new kid in town and people were curious. Where was I from? What kind of cancer did I have? How long was my treatment? There really was no question too personal to ask. It was either answer candidly or risk damaging the reputation of the "friendly Newfoundlander."

I could have stayed somewhere else of course, but the lodge was the best deal in town. Three hot meals a day and a clean bed for $70 a week. It was a cross between a hotel, a university dorm and a hospital ward. We couldn't lock our doors and we all wore identity cards around our necks, but we were free to come and go as we pleased. The lodge did have its limits though. If you were too sick to look after yourself, you couldn't stay there. The nurses regularly patrolled the rooms. One would always poke her head in at night and in the morning to make sure that I was still breathing.

"Everything okay? Any complaints?" They weren't being mother hens. A patient's condition could change dramatically, quickly. One night I saw a patient being wheeled out on a stretcher.

"Will he make it?" I asked the duty nurse.

"I think so."

All the nurses were affable, but I particularly liked Nurse Sue. Not in the Larry Flynt, fishnet-stockings, plunging-neckline, "You've been a naughty cancer patient" kind of way. No, we bonded over Bruce Springsteen. Nurse Sue was at the Springsteen concert too, and cried her eyes out when Bruce bounced into "Dancing in the Dark." That song had changed her life.

I was enraptured as she told the story. She was living in small-town England having drinks with her boyfriend at the pub. The very next day she had planned to turn down an offer to attend nursing school in Newcastle. The *Dancing in the Dark* video was on the telly. She was transfixed. The lyrics were speaking to her.

> *Man I ain't getting nowhere*
> *I'm just living in a dump like this*
> *There's something happening somewhere*
> *Baby I just know that there is*

Nurse Sue turned to her boyfriend and told him that she changed her mind about staying home, and it was all because of the video. The boyfriend was dumbfounded. "What! Because of that American bloke? We don't even know him." Sue knew enough to want a different life. She went to nursing school in far-off Newcastle, eventually dumped the boyfriend and then immigrated to Canada. Talk about a moment in time changing your life.

When I saw that Nurse Sue was hosting an Ear Nose and Throat support group meeting one evening, I went, even though I've always been jaded about such groups. I figure a friend should be able to give you the same sensible advice over a beer. My scepticism was sealed years ago when I heard about a former colleague being kicked out of his support group, after the membership had turned over twice and he still showed no signs of giving up his therapeutic crutch. Anyway, sceptics weren't welcome so I left that part of me outside the door.

I needn't have worried. This wasn't a support group in which members were encouraged to hug each other. This was an opportunity to discuss practical matters like oral hygiene. We were encouraged to use baking soda mouthwash to clear thick saliva. Timely advice, because I was starting to notice rope-like saliva in my own mouth. Gargling with a mouthwash made of one teaspoon of baking soda in two cups of water would help.

Despite being her usual bubbly self, Nurse Sue couldn't hold my attention. My mind was drifting until I heard, "Blah blah blah, screaming pain."

Whoa, what the hell was that? I thought.

"Yes, take your medication regularly so you won't wake up in the middle of the night with screaming pain. If that happens, it can take hours to get it under control."

Now, I was hanging onto Nurse Sue's every word. I learned all about the narcotics at my disposal. If codeine wasn't effective, then oxycodone or morphine could be prescribed. A cornucopia of pain relief was within grasp, enough to keep me stoned for a month. Sue assured me that I would be able to function and not get addicted, if I followed doctor's orders. And most importantly, I wouldn't be begging for mercy. I cracked the seal on the bottle of liquid codeine that night.

137

Some highs that week were natural. In keeping with my Entertainment Therapy approach I went to see Annie Lennox at Massey Hall. Her voice has always made me melt. How does a woman so white and so Scottish sound so full of soul? I would have happily walked over the broken glass she sings about to get a ticket, but that wasn't necessary. All I had to do was conduct a little seedy business with a scalper hanging around the street corner. He demanded three times the ticket price. I beat him down to two.

I was on the far right side of the fifth row. So far right that a mountain of speakers partially blocked my view, but not the part of the stage where Annie and her piano would be. The guy next to me leaned over and asked, "Same scalper?" We compared scalper prices and realized that we had been extorted equally. Perhaps there is honour among thieves after all. No matter, Annie was worth every penny. She was gorgeous. She wore a black sequined tank top that jumped off her pale skin. I couldn't take my eyes off her. And that voice. It was enchanting. Sweet dreams are made of these. Cancer just kept getting better and better.

It's Not The Food, Honest

It was a simple pappadum that brought me to my knees, metaphorically speaking. That cracker-like Indian snack, which should have been an uneventful appetizer, had me almost screaming for water in the middle of a restaurant.

The evening started well enough. I went for a run. Jogging was still part of my life though I knew I'd probably be forced to give it up sometime soon. My cousin's husband was in Toronto on a business trip and we decided to go for a trot along the waterfront after he got off work. Our route took us down Front Street past the CBC Broadcast Centre. I said nothing to Norm, but I was dreading the possibility of bumping into someone I knew.

"Glenn, what are you doing here?" would have been the natural question. I've never been good at lying.

"Me, I have this little cancer problem and I'm being irradiated for five weeks. What's new with you?" was my flippant, imaginary answer. St. John's would have heard all about it before I turned the corner. Fortunately, the awkward encounter never materialized.

I was running with a bottle of water, a concession to my dry mouth. My saliva had all but disappeared, just as every doctor, nurse, radiation therapist and brochure had predicted. The little bit of saliva that I was generating was thick. Every few minutes Norm and I slowed our strides to a fast walk. It allowed me to take a couple of quick sips, and then we picked up the pace again.

I had no trouble keeping up with Norm, as my legs were oblivious to the fact that my mouth was having a spot of bother.

A meal of Indian food was our reward for a jog well executed. A basket of pappadums was plopped on the table. I love those deep-fried wafers seasoned with cumin seeds, but I knew I'd need a little grease, so to speak, to get them down.

"May I have a mango lassie and a glass of water, please?"

"Right away, sir," said the waiter and then he rushed off to the far end of the restaurant to serve another table.

I cracked off a large piece of pappadum and started munching. I swallowed the first couple of nibbles without difficulty, but the next bits caught in the back of my throat. I needed water and I needed it now. Our waiter was nowhere in sight. Norm was chatting away, but I wasn't absorbing a single word. I tried swallowing several times. Nothing was moving down my throat. I wasn't choking; I was just terribly uncomfortable. I glanced at the bartender behind us.

"Please, I need some water right now."

He nodded yes and looked around the room for our absent waiter. His hands were busy below my sightline. The seconds dragged on. I hoped he was running the tap and getting my water. Instead, he placed a mango lassie on the bar. I thought, If that's mine I should go get it. But not wanting to appear like an impatient oaf, I didn't. I stared at the lassie. Relief was just a few feet way, but it was out of reach.

My eyes darted around the room. A second waiter was breezing past our table.

I was desperate. "Excuse me!" I raised my hands, as well as my voice. "I need some water NOW, please." I'm sure the word please was lost in the ether. There was nothing polite in my tone. He looked startled and then annoyed, but immediately brought me a glass of water. A couple of gulps and I was fine. It was a jarring scene and a tad disturbing.

"You must have been really thirsty," said Norm in the understatement of the evening.

Orillia inspired Stephen Leacock to write stories that earned him worldwide fame as a humorist. His former summer retreat is just a short stroll from Norm and Lynn's house. There is always laughter in their home and with the Stephen Leacock Museum so close, how could a cancer patient in need of a few laughs say no to an invitation for a weekend visit? As long as Lynn didn't serve pappadums with no water there'd be no trouble. At least that's what I thought.

I arrived at Lynn and Norm's house Friday afternoon able to eat most everything, albeit slowly. Lukewarm was now my favourite temperature. Milkshakes were too cold and coffee was too hot. I couldn't tolerate the extremes anymore, but everything in between was still edible. Two weeks of radiation down, three more to go. It was so far, so good.

The change was as dramatic, as it was rapid. The tipping point was Sunday dinner. Lynn had roasted a chicken, ordinarily a sumptuous meal for me. I smothered the plate in gravy, my lubricant. Everyone else at the table was raving about the meal, but to me it was awful, the worst roast chicken dinner I had ever eaten. My taste buds had completely turned against me. I twisted the peppermill over my vegetables in the hope that freshly ground pepper would give my taste buds a flavour that they liked. What a colossal mistake. It was as though I had sprinkled Scotch bonnet pepper flakes on my plate. I winced with every mouthful. It hurt. The numbing mouthwash had its limits.

I had entered the next phase of radiation side effects with stinging clarity, but I still didn't foresee the change to my bedtime routine. I went about the usual business.

1. Drink liquid codeine for pain relief.
2. Brush teeth.
3. Floss teeth.

4. Rinse with baking soda mouthwash.
5. Squirt fluoride gel into dental trays and wear for five minutes.
6. Rinse trays under tap and let air-dry thoroughly.
7. Don't rinse, eat or drink anything for one hour.

I slid under the blankets and tried to go to sleep. I felt a burning sensation creep into the back of my throat. It was concentrated on the left side, the side receiving the greatest dose of radiation, the side where they found the cancer. Perhaps I had used too much fluoride gel and the excess had slid back to the spot where my tonsil used to be. It was a slow burn. I tossed from side to side.

Don't give in, Glenn, don't give in, I said to myself. A sip of water would undo all the protection the fluoride gel was giving my teeth against tooth decay. I swallowed and swallowed and swallowed. I couldn't get the gel off the spot. The burn got hotter, it became searing. I lasted ten minutes. I couldn't take it anymore. I sipped from the glass of water on the night table. I tried not to let the water touch my teeth. I can't imagine I was very successful. I used my tongue and mouth muscles to push the water over the spot. The burning stopped. That was the last night for about a month that I used the fluoride gel.

Norm and I were on the road before sunrise. We wanted to avoid the rush-hour traffic back to Toronto. I had some green grapes and yogurt for a snack. Lynn had offered toast, but to my eyes it was a slice of sandpaper. The yogurt went down smoothly, but the grapes stung in a fashion reminiscent of the fluoride gel. It was the ascorbic acid, vitamin C. I had been warned that citrus fruits would be intolerable, but these were grapes, for God's sake. Bad enough that wine was off the menu. Now wine's mother was persona non grata as well.

Mr. President was absolutely right. He had predicted that my sore throat would appear by Monday and appear it did, in all its glory. With that kind of insight, Mr. President should have been in The White House.

The folks at the Princess Margaret Hospital Lodge didn't really know how to handle a resident like me. Almost everyone else could eat normally. The food line served three hot meals a day, but these were meals for people who didn't have a raw throat. Pasta could still slither down, but very little else in solid food was tolerable. Soft eggs, puddings, Jell-O and Cream of Wheat became my staples. Sometimes, I found myself staring at the menu board, only to realize that there was nothing on it that I could eat.

The blue star on my identification tag meant that I was allowed extra goodies, such as meal replacement drinks. The ladies behind the counter seemed to have interpreted the star to mean that I should be offered an extra large serving of beef on a bun with my French fries. A nice gesture, but without the whole works going into a blender, it was off limits. The staff probably would have given it a whirl had I asked, but the thought wasn't very appetizing.

I started drinking the odd container of Boost, which I bought at the drugstore I passed every day. The packaging promised a bounty of protein, vitamins and anti-oxidants, but the only thing I was really interested in were the calories. I could get 360 calories per bottle. The lodge's meal replacement drink had only 250 calories. It was no contest. I figured I had only so many swallows, so I should get the biggest bang for my buck.

The phrase six-pack took on a whole new meaning.

Nurse Terry wasn't kidding when she said that Princess Margaret Hospital Lodge was in the gay neighbourhood. Church Street was lined with porn shops, leather bars and bathhouses. And while I've had experience getting naked and soaped up with strange men, I wasn't tempted to go inside.

You see my experience with "bathhouses" was in Japan, where

they are very big on the bathing part and not at all big on the sex part. The Japanese onsen is a public bath that has tapped into a hot spring. One of the few pluses to living in a volcanic region. The onsen is open to couples, families and friends. An onsen can be inside or outside, and is a place to relax and socialize. The water is blistering hot, often 40 degrees centigrade. Onsens are heavenly.

The cardinal rule of any onsen is that you must scrub down *before* you slip into the steaming-hot pool. Not washing beforehand is taboo. The actual washing is a bit silly looking. Big men sitting on stools sized for five-year-old children, using hand showers, trying not to splash the neighbours. You wander into the bath with a modesty cloth strategically held in front of the naughty bits, even though the sexes are segregated. The payoff is wonderful. All aches and pains are soaked away.

I loved onsens, even after I nearly had a heart attack in one. I was at a ski resort in Hokkaido and had just come inside after simmering in a light snowfall. I was buck-naked in the change room, my modesty cloth tossed into the laundry bin. I spun around and came face-to-face with a cleaning lady. I blurted out, "Sumimasen" (*Excuse me*), bowed and scrunched together. She, on the other hand, was completely nonchalant. I realized that she had actually averted her eyes.

The cleaning lady was in the change room every time I was there afterwards. Her head was never up. It must be odd to spend a good portion of your day staring at the floor, but she did it. It was as though she didn't exist. Japanese culture allowed me to stand in my birthday suit next to a grandmotherly woman and not be embarrassed. What a country!

You can never run from your past. Well, it wasn't so much my past as my province's past. One of the residents at the lodge was a former deputy fire marshal in Ontario. Over lunch he told me that a highlight of his career was re-investigating a suspicious fire in a former Newfoundland cabinet minister's apartment.

Tom Farrell's name still sends a shudder through the CBC legal department. In the late 1970s, the CBC broadcast that Farrell deliberately set fire to his apartment. The story was based on a leaked and flawed police report. Farrell successfully sued the CBC for $50,000 because CBC couldn't prove the allegation.

Alan and his colleagues at the Ontario fire marshal's office re-created the fire scene, and found no crime.

Having established that the Newfoundland investigators of the day were imperfect, Alan turned his attention to corruption in my home province.

"One of the sergeants who investigated Mount Cashel Orphanage told me that the chief of police told him to change his report."

Suddenly, I felt small. Alan knew all about the pedophile Christian Brothers and the cover-up. What was there to do except express shock and disgust at the police officers and justice officials who betrayed their oath, and the boys. The child abuse revelations were sickening. There is no way to calculate the damage done, the lives destroyed.

Awkward silence. I struggled to get down a few forkfuls of food. "Now," said Alan, "what happened to the Indians in Newfoundland?"

If I were in Japan right now, I thought, the earth might open up and save me from this torment, but noooo, I'm stuck in Ontario with no chance of an earthquake.

The extinction of the Beothuk is an awful and bloody chapter in our history. They starved to death after losing access to the coast or were hunted down in reprisal killings. The only good spin I've ever heard about the Beothuk's demise came from the comedy troupe Codco. They had a sketch in which an indignant Newfoundlander explained to a pious mainlander that the Beothuk were a very skittish people, and we only shot them to stop them from running away.

I don't think Alan meant to make me squirm. He was just

making conversation. That's what he knew about Newfoundland — scandals and moments of infamy.

He was Basil Fawlty and I was the Germans. Please Alan, next time, don't mention the war.

Norm and I jogged past Rogers Centre, home of the Toronto Blue Jays. Baseball wasn't on my Entertainment Therapy agenda; it was the wrong time of the year. No matter, I had plenty of baseball memories from Japan to daydream about.

The Tokyo Dome is every bit as impressive as the Rogers Centre. Murakami-san managed against great odds to buy tickets to a Saturday afternoon game. Deb and I met him and his baby daughter outside the Dome. Murakami-san sat little Sakura by Deb and said, "New mother." We went to get beer and burgers.

Murakami-san was always fun company, even at work. If I heard "Glenn-san, I need your power," Murakami-san needed me to decipher some videotape where the English speaker had a thick accent. Once, the troublesome word was "absolutely." I scrawled it on a piece of paper. Thanks to my bad penmanship and a spelling mistake, poor Murakami-san spent the next five minutes with his nose in a dictionary, trying to figure out what the hell I had written. When he finally did, he said, "We will sign up for English lessons together."

The Yomiuri Giants were playing the Rakuten Golden Eagles. The Giants are the New York Yankees of Japan. They are the wealthiest, oldest, most-popular team in the Japanese pro league, and they've won more championships than any other team.

Notice that they're not called the Tokyo Giants. Yomiuri is a newspaper conglomerate. Rakuten is an Internet shopping mall. Baseball teams in Japan are marketing tools for the companies that own them. My favourite moniker is the Nippon Ham Fighters. Just as the name implies, they're owned by a meat packing company.

Frankly, it's against my nature to cheer for capitalist greed. "Come on, shopping mall, ring up my credit card." It just doesn't flow off my lips. But clearly, I was the only one troubled by the nomenclature. There were 50,000 fans in the Dome and they had no hesitation in cheering.

The bleacher creatures were the most fun to watch. There were horns and drums, banners and flags, and chants. Relentless chanting. They didn't shut up for the entire nine innings. But it was all orchestrated and choreographed. The group cheered, not individuals. No one heckled. This was polite cheering. This was Japanese cheering. It wouldn't work on our side of the pond.

By the end of the week, Norm was probably thinking that he should never invite me out to dinner again.

Norm suggested a vegan restaurant that he had heard featured on CBC radio. Despite my love of all things on the hoof, I've been known to enjoy the odd vegetarian meal, so we set out for the Urban Herbivore in Kensington Market. It had a reputation for creamy hearty soups, and that seemed just the ticket for a guy unable to swallow much solid food.

We found a parking spot half a block away. I used the privacy of the car to carry out my pre-meal ritual. I needed to swish the numbing mouthwash around my mouth. I was carrying a tablespoonful in a urine specimen bottle, a *sterile* urine specimen bottle. Yes, I checked to see if the seal had been broken beforehand. The nurses at the lodge had given me several bottles for occasions just like this. I could leave the big medicine bottle in my room and discreetly carry a pre-measured amount.

The trick was to swish the mouthwash for one minute, about ten minutes before eating. That would allow time for the optimum numbing effect. The numbness lasted about twenty-five minutes, time enough to get my food down. The medical information sheet warned that the numbing might increase the danger of accidentally biting my cheeks or tongue, so I should chew slowly. I wouldn't be chewing my soup, so nothing could possibly go wrong.

I had the option of swishing and spitting, or swishing and swallowing, up to four times a day. Spit or swallow? Such debates usually have a bawdy connotation, complete with smirks and snickers. Having no experience in these matters, I was free to choose my own path. Early on, I decided that I was a swallow man. A good thing too. It was hard to be otherwise sitting in Norm's car.

The Urban Herbivore was brimming with a wonderful curry aroma. I ordered a bowl of leek and potato soup. I had just spoken the words when I felt my stomach churn. This was no time to scamper to the bathroom only to discover that it was already occupied. I ran outside and promptly threw up in the plants, several times. As a culinary statement, this was extreme, even for me. I kept thinking I should tell passers-by, "It's not the food, honest, it's me."

Norm came out to check on me. "I cancelled your order."

Let this be a warning to all vegetarian restaurants: don't let Glenn Deir darken your door.

"There's no screwing around here." Naoto's email made me laugh out loud. His use of that phrase always made me laugh out loud.

The joke dated back to a script that Naoto had once filed for my approval. Japan was getting increasingly annoyed at North Korea's boycott of negotiations aimed at having the North abandon nuclear research in exchange for food and energy aid. Japan was floating the idea of sanctions. Naoto translated the admonition from the Japanese foreign ministry spokesman as, "We're not screwing around here."

I had a belly laugh and Naoto looked mortified. I had wounded his pride by laughing at his English. He had lost face. It was a terrible transgression on my part, unintentional, but a transgression nonetheless. I apologized for causing him embarrassment, and explained that the phrase was slang and best used among friends and colleagues. I delved into the nuance of the expression, that screwing around could mean one is sexually promiscuous or one is fooling around wasting time. Naoto smiled. The foreign ministry spokesman obviously wanted to convey Japan's impatience with North Korea. I suggested a better translation might be, "We're fed up and we're serious about sanctions." Naoto agreed. For months afterwards though, he'd use our private conversations to drop in the phrase "I'm not screwing around here."

Naoto had seen an email I sent Susumu, outlining my medical problems. He knew about the lump in my neck and the early theory that it might be an infection I had picked up in Japan. Perhaps Naoto now thought I had picked up cancer there instead. He wrote, "Thank you for educating me. I had to consult the dictionary more than ten times to read through your medical report ... Everything has an end. I believe you have the power to overcome the gift from Japan. There's no screwing around here."

Naoto and my other friends at NHK World taught me a great deal about the nuances of the Japanese language. One of my proudest moments came when I made a joke in Nihongo, which is Japanese for Japanese.

It came at the expense of Japan's soldiers in Iraq, though I wasn't allowed to call the soldiers *soldiers* in any NHK script. They were *troops* or *military personnel*. And they were not in the army. They were in the Ground Self-Defense Force. Japan's constitution renounces war, so the country is not legally allowed to have an army. The fact that Japan's *soldiers* run around in uniforms, carry weapons and are trained to kill doesn't matter. This was a war of words I could not win.

Omura-san and I were discussing what words we should superimpose over video of Japanese troops leaving Iraq after two years. The Ground Self-Defense Force had been kept far from the fighting and spent much of its time doing reconstruction work like building roads. By July 2006, the mission was over and the military personnel were coming home.

Omura-san wondered about using Sayonara as our written banner. I assured her that Sayonara had no negative connotation in English and that many English speakers would recognize it as a Japanese word for goodbye.

Then the Evil Glenn spoke up. "Maybe we should say, Osakini shitsurei shimasu." Omura-san and several others burst out laughing. Get it! Osakini shitsurei shimasu. Hello! Anybody out there? Is this mic on? Tough crowd.

All right, here's the joke. The Japanese have about a dozen ways to say goodbye. It depends on the social context. Osakini shitsurei shimasu is sometimes used at the office. It means, *Pardon my rudeness for leaving before you have finished your work.* Japan was pulling out of Iraq by itself, leaving other countries behind to finish the job of getting Iraq back on its feet. Now do you get it? You're probably thinking, Keep your day job, Glenn. But trust me; this joke kills them in Tokyo.

Dr. Maxymiw's dental chair felt like a confessional. I had to confess my sins and I'm not even Catholic.

"I stopped using the dental trays. The fluoride gel was burning my throat."

"People always use too much," said Dr. Maxymiw. "Use only a couple of drops and spread them around with a Q-tip."

"I tried. It still burns too much."

"If you have to give them up for a while, that's okay. Start using them again as soon as you can."

I was full of complaints. "I can't seem to find a toothbrush that's soft enough." I had a blister on the inside of my lower lip and no matter how careful I was, I always managed to stab it with a bristle. It hurt like hell.

"Try this one," said Dr. Maxymiw as he handed me a toothbrush with extra soft bristles.

"Open wide." Opening wide was no longer an option. And neither were proper chewing and speaking properly. The radiation had caused my jaw muscles to tighten. I certainly didn't look or sound like a guy who made his living as a television reporter.

"Have you started taking your liquid codeine yet?" asked Dr. Waldron.

I had been, of course, ever since Nurse Sue gave me the lecture about avoiding screaming pain. Every four hours, I faithfully measured five millilitres into a medicine cup and tossed it back. Five millilitres was half the amount I was allowed to consume. I was following Nurse Sue's advice to give myself a little wiggle room for when the side effects got worse.

I was just taking in a breath to answer Dr. Waldron when he said, "Don't bother, I can tell by your eyes."

I had no pain. But I was walking around stoned, and looked it. An acceptable trade-off. Just call me Doper Deir.

Dr. Waldron glanced at my chart and he didn't look pleased. I had lost six pounds since our meeting a week ago. "I don't want to give you a G-tube, but ..." He didn't have to finish the sentence. I got the message. Buck up, or it's surgery for you, my little St. John's friend. I thought I had put a stake through the heart of the dreaded gastrostomy, but no, the feeding tube had become a stick and I was being hit with it.

The carrot was to consume more calories and stem the weight loss, or at least slow it down. Eating more soft food was out of the question. I could barely get down the little bit on my plate already. I'd have to pick up the pace on the meal replacement drinks. If I could get three of them down a day, plus a little food, I might avoid that bloated feeling which comes from having a feeding tube sticking out of your stomach.

Variety was an enemy. Boost was my meal replacement drink of choice and it came in only three flavours: strawberry, vanilla and chocolate. Ordinarily, I adore chocolate, but the laxative syrup I was taking came with a chocolate flavour. I suddenly lost my taste for chocolate Boost. I was left with alternating between the two other flavours. If I had strawberry for breakfast, then it would be vanilla for lunch. Yum, yum.

What was that tune? It was driving me crazy. I knew it, but couldn't name it. All patients were welcome to relax to their own music during treatment, but I always let the radiation therapists pick out the CD. The same jazzy instrumental music had been playing for several days. I couldn't take it any longer.

"Do you mind if I look at the CD?" I said after hopping down from the table.

"Anything wrong?"

"Oh no. I just can't remember the name of one of the songs."

It was a burned CD, with no song list. Beegie Adair Trio was written in felt pen. Never heard of them.

When I got back to the lodge I did a little Google research. The answer to the mystery made me laugh out loud. The tune that had been driving me crazy was Frank Sinatra's "I Get A Kick Out Of You." This absurd moment brought to you by cancer, again.

> I get no kick from champagne
> Mere alcohol doesn't thrill me at all
> So tell me why should it be true
> That I get a kick out of you

The twisted irony was far more delicious than anything I was eating. I was delighted when it was still on the CD player the next day. I was wearing a big grin underneath the mask.

Sleep Demon

I came to with a snort.

I couldn't believe it. I started week four of my treatment by actually falling asleep on the table as the radiation machine was growling around me. You'd think that I could stay awake for fifteen minutes, but a wave washed over me and I was filling the room with Zs. I was only out a minute or so, but I realized when I woke up that my jaw was slack, allowing my mouth to droop a little. I was alarmed because radiation calculations are precise and you're not supposed to move. I remembered the three-millimetre threshold for error. It seemed to me that my mouth was open more than three millimetres. I wondered if some part of my mouth had gotten more than its prescribed share of radiation.

The immobilization mask was designed to hold me together and down, but weight loss had made my face slimmer and there was a little slack underneath the Ghostly Glenn. Lose too much weight and I'd need another mask. The radiation therapists seemed more concerned about my thinning face than my napping. Some people are so on edge during radiation that merely passing the immobilization mask over their faces can set off an anxiety attack. But I was able to snore away, seemingly without empathy for their plight.

As the week went on, the Sleep Demon became my constant companion. The Sleep Demon is the cancer version of the

Sandman. Instead of sprinkling magic dust in my eyes, the Sleep Demon used high-energy x-rays to lull me to sleep. He didn't have the slightest regard for the time of day, or circumstances.

I was chronically tired by the time brother-in-law Steve landed in Toronto, just as I feared back in Christian's Bar in St. John's. I'd wake up to have breakfast, only to lie down again afterwards for a nap until it was time to walk to the hospital for treatment. To make matters worse, my clenched jaw and swollen tongue made normal speech impossible. I simply couldn't shape words properly. Still, Steve was charitable in his assessment, albeit with a backhanded compliment.

"You don't look as bad as I thought you'd be."

I was glad to see him. I had gone through a couple of room-mates and while they were pleasant company, they weren't friends. The lodge allowed a friend or relative to stay in a room, as long as a cancer patient didn't need the bed. The lodge was below capacity that week so Steve was welcome.

Steve had embraced my notion of Entertainment Therapy; insisted on it, in fact. There'd be no lounging around the room telling woe-is-me tales. First on the itinerary was a concert by The Waterboys, an Irish/Scottish band, best known in my neck of the woods for the song "Bang on the Ear."

Unfortunately for me, the Sleep Demon made an unwelcome appearance at the Danforth Music Hall. It tapped me on the shoulder and when I turned around to look, it hit me with a 2 by 4. What a bang on the ear! I knew I was in trouble when I started swaying, but not in time with the music. I was in danger of top-pling over the drunken Irish/Scottish wannabees standing in front of me. That seemed like a sure way to start an epic row.

"I've got to go. I can barely stand up."

The concert was just half over. Steve offered to take me back to the room, but I declined.

"You stay and enjoy the show. I'll be all right."

I was facing a fifteen-minute subway ride. How could I avoid sleeping through my stop? I needed to be Japanese more than ever. A Japanese has the remarkable and handy ability to sleep soundly upright and wake up just as the train is pulling into his station. I saw it dozens of times.

Frequently, it involved a salaryman, presumably after a long day at the office, with his head flopped over on the shoulder of the person sitting next to him. The put-upon passenger would never wake up the snoozing salaryman or try to shrug the head in the other direction. The practice was so common that even gaijin (foreigners) were granted the privilege. Once, on a train to Nikko, I spied an East Indian man sound asleep with his head resting on the shoulder of a Japanese man. The Japanese looked straight ahead, as if nothing untoward were happening.

It was an infectious habit, and never more apparent than when Deb and I were taking an early morning train down the peninsula that divides Tokyo Bay. We were on our way to see a thirty-one metre high Buddha on a mountaintop. Instead of using the time to contemplate the true meaning of life, I was tormenting Deb. She had told me about meeting a friend's "friend" who was handy in the kitchen. I suspected he had skill in another room of the apartment. I shamelessly stole lines from the Monty Python comedy team.

"Likes to cook, does he? Know what I mean. Nudge, nudge. Know what I mean. Wink's as good as a nod to a blind man."

Deb was fed up. "Shhhhh! People are trying to sleep." I glanced around and noticed that every other head in the car was bouncing up and down with the rocking of the train.

To the best of my memory, I didn't let my head flop on anyone's shoulder on the way back to the lodge. And while I drifted off to sleep for a stop or two, I managed to fend off the Sleep Demon long enough to get off at Wellesley Station. I was in another dimension when Steve came in through the door.

Steve and I said, "Damn the torpedoes, full speed ahead." Tuesday night was *We Will Rock You*, a show based on the music of Queen.

It wasn't high theatre, but it sure was fun. We were bobbing our heads during "Bohemian Rhapsody," and neither of us was falling asleep.

The piece de résistance of Steve's week of caregiving was a big-league basketball game — Toronto Raptors vs. Orlando Magic. Steve had arranged for tickets just five rows back from the court, practically underneath a basket. Close enough to see every swinging elbow in the mad scramble to grab a rebound.

I went into the Air Canada Centre more interested in the spectacle than the actual game, but the game turned out to be quite entertaining. Toronto almost pulled it out of the fire, getting the lead for the first time with just a few minutes left. But Orlando held its ground and went on to win 105 — 96.

No insult intended, but basketball players aren't normal. In size, that is. They all look about two feet taller than I am, and I'm 6'1". They're great athletes though. No argument from me. I learned in Japan not to doubt athletic prowess because of freakish size. Sumo wrestlers, I came to realize, are not fat slobs. They are great athletes too — skilled, strong, agile.

Deb and I spent a morning at the Azumazeki Beya stable watching the wrestlers train. Stable is the perfect word because sumo wrestlers are treated like prized horses. They're corralled together and groomed for success.

The Azumazeki Beya stable-master is a legend in Japan. Jesse Kuhaulua originally came from Hawaii and was the first non-Japanese to win a Grand Sumo Tournament. He was a giant of a man in his prime — 6' 4" and over 450 pounds.

Kuhaulua-san has a raspy voice and cauliflower ears, the ears being the product of innumerable body slams and wrestling holds. The stable is his retirement business. There was no doubt about who was in charge. When the master spoke, everyone leapt to attention, perhaps because if they didn't, they might get a whack from the "motivation" stick that sat within arm's reach.

We had the honour of sitting just behind Kuhaulua-san during practice, which was a bit of a problem actually, because he's lost none of his bulk since retirement. I spent a lot of time leaning to the side or craning my neck. The view only got worse when a large grey poodle plopped down by Kuhaulua-san and on my feet. I goosed it a few times with my toes, but it wouldn't budge. I suffered in silence. One does not complain in a sumo stable. One endures.

I've never seen so many taped-up ankles, toes, fingers, wrists, knees and elbows. Only a handful of the wrestlers didn't have something injured. After watching them work out, I'm not surprised. What you don't hear on television, or in the upper deck of the sumo arena, is the thunderous wallop when they slam into each other. The training is gruelling. They fight bout after bout, to the point of exhaustion.

The winner chooses his opponent. The instant a practice fight is over, the underlings on the edge of the ring put up their hands and yell, "Pick me, pick me!" A wrestler can't advance unless he gets noticed, and he can't get noticed unless he fights. And wins.

The star wrestler at the stable was Takamisakari, ranked fifteenth best in the country at the time. The fans love him. His nickname is Robocop because he walks with a choppy stride. He's a growler and a grunter, who likes to slap his waist louder than all the other wrestlers.

Takamisakari was having a bad morning. The growling and grunting got more ferocious as a young buck continuously beat him. Finally, Takamisakari drove the upstart across the ring and slammed him into a wall. He let out a moan as he crumpled.

I could never be a sumo wrestler, and not because of the threat of injury or pain. After all, I took a bit of punishment in my hockey playing days, including a broken nose. The body slams alone didn't scare me off. No, what convinced me that I don't have the right stuff to step into the ring was a moment of servitude. Takamisakari hawked into a tissue and nonchalantly dropped it into the hand of a junior wrestler, who unflinchingly carried it over to the trashcan.

"Don't pick me, don't pick me," I said to myself.

"I heard," said the nurse, "that Newfoundland is very beautiful."

I started to laugh.

"No, really, my sister has been there and she loved it."

I didn't quarrel with the nurse's impression of Newfoundland, or her sister's. My laughter had all to do with the absurd situation for such small talk. You see, I was bent over a bathroom sink receiving an enema. It had been a week since I had been regular, shall we say. I didn't even have the desire to use the toilet, but I knew seven days without a bowel movement was not good for my health, and the nurses at the Radiation Nursing Clinic knew it too.

"I'm going to squeeze in some liquid and you hold it for as long as you can before letting go," the nurse added.

The codeine that was protecting me from screaming pain had my intestines tied in a knot. My constipation was a prophecy come true. It was a shock to no one, least of all me. The comings and goings of my gastrointestinal tract had become a favourite topic amongst nurses at the lodge and radiation therapists at the hospital. They wanted me to have a bowel movement at least once every three days. I was way overdue.

The bowel report was a favourite topic of Room 413's morning banter. Put two guys in something that resembles a university dorm and I think it's inevitable that toilet humour will rear its juvenile head. Steve fretted that my insides might go septic if I didn't go to the bathroom soon. I shot back that maybe someone else could use the toilet, if only he would vacate it. All of which culminated with a Newfoundland travel tips conversation with a nurse as she deftly negotiated a hose past the cutest cheeks in the bathroom.

Operation Dam Buster was a success. And to ensure that it wasn't repeated, the nurses put me on mega doses of stool softeners and laxatives, everything I needed to keep the river free of logjams.

"If the cancer is going to recur, it usually happens in the first twelve to eighteen months," said Dr. Waldron. I still had another six treatments to go, but Dr. Waldron was already tying off loose ends and getting ready to say goodbye.

"I'd like a CT scan three months after the end of treatment, to give us a baseline once the swelling goes down. Some follow-up is required every two or three months for the next two years."

"I'll tell my doctors in St. John's."

"I close my file on you in five years."

Five years is frequently the magic number you hear associated with cancer. Five years cancer-free, and you're considered cured.

"Dr. Waldron, how many gray am I getting on my throat?" Radiation is measured in units called gray, abbreviated Gy. It's named after Louis Harold Gray, a British scientist. Gray devoted much of his life's research to understanding how to effectively use irradiation to destroy cancerous cells while sparing nearby healthy tissue.

Dr. Waldron took his pen and started drawing on the tissue paper covering the examination table. A round head, round eyes, a horseshoe nose, a neck, a chest, and a couple of arms. He sketched four small oval shapes on the paper man's cheeks and neck, and then amoeba shapes around those.

"This is not the exact pattern," he said, pointing to the egg-like shapes, "but these areas are getting 60 gray over twenty-five days. The larger areas receive 50 gray."

My heart sank: 60 gray was not what I was hoping to hear. Salivary glands exposed to doses larger than 54 gray suffer irreversible damage. Dr. Deir matched the oval shapes with his rudimentary knowledge of where the salivary glands are located. It was Dr. Deir's Internet-educated opinion that the prognosis was grim. Dr. Waldron's ovals were hovering dangerously near the parotid glands. We have two of them, one per cheek under the ear. The parotid glands produce more saliva than any others, and are more susceptible to radiation damage than any others. The medical literature was very clear. If my parotid glands were receiving 60 gray, they were as good as dead.

But there was a glimmer of hope for the others. The salivary glands underneath my tongue were in the 50 gray or less zone. They might have some function afterwards, and perhaps even compensate for the lack of saliva from the parotid glands. My saliva had all but disappeared. How much it would recover was really anyone's guess.

As I fretted about spit in Toronto, there was profound discomfort in Comfort Cove. My sister's house burned down. Barb and her husband Ted escaped unharmed, but they got out with only the clothes on their backs. By the time the Comfort Cove Volunteer Fire Department got their hoses turned on, the house was engulfed in flames. Everything was lost.

Barb told me that she was inside the house when the fire broke out. She didn't even know it was happening. Ted was outside puttering around the shed when he saw the smoke. He raced back into the house and roared at Barb to get out. The flames broke through shortly afterwards.

Investigators determined the source of the fire was an electrical fault. Barb and Ted had insurance, and they were promised a new home in the spring. Barb said they were fine. They would stay with Ted's sister until they could find a house to rent.

Barb was burned out of her house. I was fighting cancer. Fate had no lack of imagination when designing misfortune for the Deir siblings.

I was fighting my own version of morning sickness. Sometimes, the thought of eating early in the day made my stomach queasy.

I had to quell the sensation before attempting eggs or anything else. A single egg could take half an hour to get down. I was finding it increasingly difficult to swallow, but balked at some suggestions.

"Try some butter on your eggs," said Steve.

"I don't like butter."

"It will help you get them down."

"I don't like butter."

I punctuated the mouthfuls of food with a cocktail made of Boost and whole milk. Half and half was the best blend. Before starting radiation treatment, I always drank one per cent milk and very little of it, usually just on cereal. I wanted to avoid calories then, but now I needed all the calories I could get.

I experimented unsuccessfully with a variety of smoothie drinks from the grocery store. No matter what the fruit, I couldn't tolerate the acid. Mango, kiwi, strawberry, it didn't matter. One sip and I'd wince. I even tried baby food, but it also set off reverberations of stinging.

I had virtually no chewing ability left. I found food particles were getting caught under my tongue and it was like grit. I couldn't clear them without a great deal of water-swishing. Egg salad, with its small bits of onion and sweet pepper, was no longer a good choice. Cottage cheese was a chore, so I gave up that too.

One evening, Steve and I abandoned the lodge's cafeteria and we ducked into a Marriott hotel on Yonge Street. I foolishly ordered a shrimp and pasta dish.

"I know this may sound odd, but would you please ask the chef to put the meal into a blender and blend it up," I said to the waiter, finally trying what I never asked the staff at the lodge to do. "I have a very sore throat and can't swallow easily. Oh, no pepper or spices please."

The chef did exactly as I asked. The pasta and shrimp came to the table as a congealed blob, about as inviting as plasterer's mud. I took a forkful and felt burning all around my mouth. I guess the chef ignored the bit about no pepper. I laid the fork on the plate.

"I can't eat it."

Steve finished his meal. I didn't attempt another bite.

I admit that I can be a bit prickly sometimes, but I thought cancer had taken the edge off. I was wrong.

The flash point happened during a support group meeting for people fighting head and neck cancers. The nurse didn't recognize one guy. When she asked who he was, he said, "Oh, I've got prostate cancer. I was wondering if I could stay and see how these things work." No one had any objections and we dove into the minutiae of our problems.

Many of us had dry lips. I took a tube of lip balm out of my pocket.

"This has worked for me," I said, holding up the Lypsyl. "It's Aloha flavour." There were chuckles around the circle.

"The radiation therapist checked the ingredients and said it was okay. Don't put it on before treatment though. Apparently it can change the way the radiation passes through the skin." A couple of people asked to see the tube.

The discussion turned to meal replacement drinks. There was a debate about which one gives you the most calories in the least number of swallows. Mr. Prostate Cancer piped up. "Hey, I don't know, but I heard you can have a tube put down your throat and you can pour food in through a funnel."

Everyone went stony silent. At this stage most of us would have had exhaustive discussions with our doctors about the pros and cons of feeding tubes. For all I knew, someone in the room might have had one sticking out of his stomach, neatly hidden under a shirt. In that moment, Mr. Prostate Cancer crystallized into all the instant experts I had endured since testing positive for cancer, the instant experts who were compelled to pass along all information, no matter how outrageous, irrelevant or untrue.

Until then, I accepted it all graciously. Most often it was a reflection of people's nervousness and a desire to say something encouraging.

Mr. Prostate Cancer should have known better. I put as much steel into my eyes and voice as I could muster and said, "This … is … not … helpful."

He never uttered another peep for the rest of the meeting. Later, we met by the cafeteria menu, both of us staring at the evening's choices, while I held on to my bottle of Boost.

"Pizza looks good," he said as he walked inside.

Allan Gardens is the closest green oasis to the lodge, and that's where Steve and I were headed as we jogged down Jarvis Street. I had a bottle of water slipped into a holster in the small of my back. It was a sunny, cool day — perfect running weather. The gardens were gorgeous. We trotted around the greenhouses and fountain at an easy pace.

I had been a runner for twenty years, but I knew my time was up. It made no sense to burn off calories that I couldn't afford to lose. I wasn't consuming enough calories to maintain my weight, and there was no hope that I could increase my food intake in the foreseeable future. And then there was the fatigue. I felt like I was carrying the Sleep Demon on my back. I didn't have the energy anymore.

There was a time I hated jogging, but it evolved into an activity that I looked forward to. Never more so than in Tokyo. Every jog brought the possibility of a Tokyo snapshot, a slice of Tokyo life that I hadn't seen before.

Yoyogi Park was a favourite destination for long runs. That's where I saw actors rehearsing their parts. The one pretending to wash his laundry was berating the one wearing the surgical mask. I doubt the mask was a prop. At the first sign of a cold, Tokyoites wear surgical masks to prevent spreading their germs. Taking a day off work and staying home until the sniffles stop is not the

Japanese way. If the actor did wear the mask on stage, a Japanese audience wouldn't blink an eye. It's part of everyday life. I frequently had conversations at NHK where my colleagues were speaking through gauze.

Sometimes the Evil Glenn shows up when I least expect him. Dozens of blind joggers in Yoyogi Park brought him out one day. Each was paired with a guide, and they were connected by a loop of rope in their hands. Some were running at a pretty good clip, as fast as me. I thought, Such courage, such trust.

Then admiration turned into snickering. I blame Codco, that Newfoundland comedy troupe which gave me a lifetime of politically incorrect humour. I remembered a sketch about a taxi from around the bay headed to St. John's. One of the passengers is blind and when the others discover this, they shout at him as if he were deaf. They say the most condescending things, such as, "It must be awful being a burden to everybody." Of course the blind man denies this, saying he can do most things for himself. The condescending passengers won't give up. "Oh, I know you can do the blind things. But you can't get married or anything like that."

The Evil Glenn was shouting at the blind joggers inside my head. Oh, I know you can do the blind things. But you can't run or anything like that.

I'm sure a particularly hot corner of hell has been reserved for me.

Jogging through Tokyo taught me that despite having the second largest economy in the world, Japan does have its destitute and its homeless. One woman in particular stood out. We were neighbours, kind of. I lived in a nice apartment in Shangri-la; she lived on a park bench at the end of the street. I saw her every time I jogged the promenade, went to the grocery store, picked up a video, or took the subway. That meant I saw her just about every day.

All her worldly possessions were in plastic bags sitting around her or neatly stacked on a cart. I often wondered about her background. I never saw her with drugs or alcohol. She didn't bay at the moon. She took pride in her appearance, regularly changing her clothes. She took pride in the appearance of her "home" too. She used to sweep up the leaves around the park bench. I always made a point of giving her a wide berth whenever I jogged by. I could never shake the feeling that I was running through her living room. She smiled when we made eye contact and we exchanged hellos, but my Japanese didn't allow for anthropological conversations.

I saw a kind-hearted person giving her a poncho, just in time for the deluge that night. During typhoon season, she occasionally escaped the horizontal rain by slipping inside the subway station.

She spent countless hours on the park bench watching the world pass her by. She slept there, too, though not very comfortably, I'm sure. The bench had a divider, making it impossible to stretch out. Her legs either hung off the end or she slept sitting up. I read in Donald Richie's book, *The Japan Journals,* that the benches were deliberately designed with a divider to discourage occupancy by the homeless.

One morning she was gone. A few days later, so were her park bench and the nearby metal barricades she used as a clothesline. Now that's an eviction notice. Weeks later she reappeared farther down the promenade, again taking up residence on a park bench. She didn't seem to have as many bags this time. She didn't smile and looked much sadder. Life had kicked her again.

Winter was fast approaching and the temperature slipped below freezing at night. She wrapped a scarf around her head, making her look like a Russian babushka. One frosty morning she was rubbing her shoeless foot to bring back the circulation. Ten minutes later, I jogged by again and she was rubbing the other foot. There are hundreds, if not thousands, like her in Tokyo.

I saw no homeless in Toronto's Allan Gardens. No one to make me feel guilty about my good fortune in life. It was a splendid location for a finale. Steve and I ended the run with a sprint in front of the lodge. I would not jog again for eight months.

It was a tad demoralizing to walk into a bar and order a glass of milk, but that didn't stop me from doing it a few times during radiation treatment. Steve celebrated his birthday while he was in Toronto, and it didn't seem right not to go out for a drink, even though I couldn't drink alcohol. Norm was in town again on business, and he led us to a bar that specialized in beer from around the world. The waitress had the decency not to scoff at my order. And she didn't charge a corkage fee when I opened my Boost. Maybe people order milk in bars all the time. But I felt foolish, as if I shouldn't be wasting her time if alcohol wasn't going to appear on the bill.

Another day Steve and I had finished a little Christmas shopping (I picked up a headlamp for Deb's stocking, for the next time we hike up Fuji-san) when we spied that bastion of male lechery disguising itself as a family restaurant — Hooters. I was fairly certain that seeing beautiful women in orange shorts and tank tops was not a cure for cancer, but just in case I was wrong, we swaggered in. Steve ordered a beer and food, and I brought out the Boost and ordered a glass of milk.

"Put mine in a dirty glass," I added. It got a laugh from the waitress. I still had it.

Graduation Day

I joked with Steve that I had to send him back to St. John's so I could finally get some rest. My dance card had been full all week and despite the fatigue, staying active was the right thing to do. There were times I forgot how sick I was. Twenty treatments down, five more to go. Deb would be with me for the home stretch.

While radiation therapy was ploughing on, the curtain was dropping on my Entertainment Therapy. I had spoken to Deb over the phone about us taking in a hockey game. This was a gamble because Deb really doesn't like the sport.

"Honey, the Canadiens are playing the Leafs. It doesn't get more Canadian than that."

Silence. Long silence. Really long silence. Deb cleared her throat. "I'll go if you want me to."

There are times in a husband's life when "Yes" means "No" and I figured this was one of those times. My salivary glands might be dead, but my brain wasn't.

Deb flew in Saturday morning and I met her at the airport. It felt good to give her a hug. A long passionate kiss was out of the question. My throat and mouth had changed quite a bit since she had last seen me. The side effects of radiation treatment had blossomed. Clenched teeth, swollen tongue, red skin, blister on the inside lower lip — the new me would take some getting used to.

However, Deb was not so overcome with anxiety that she stopped herself from poking fun at me. I reminded her of a Maori wrasse we saw while snorkelling on the Great Barrier Reef in Australia. It's a giant fish, about six feet long, with a prominent hump on its head and thick lips. I guess Deb saw a resemblance in the thick lips.

"Oh, my little wrasse," she said while touching my cheek. "If a wrasse could talk, it would sound just like you."

I sounded like I had a giant jawbreaker in my mouth. I had only one defence, play the cancer card. "I've got cancer and you're making fun of me?"

Nothing like a pity-inducing retort to win the day. This was going to be a good week, even if I didn't get to see the Leafs and Canadiens.

Kurt had kindly driven down from Hamilton to scoop us up. He and my cousin Ann were once again willing to take in the Newfoundland waifs and strays for the weekend.

I spent most of Saturday and Sunday napping. My goal each night was to stay up until nine o'clock. Ann, Kurt and Deb went off to a concert Sunday evening without me, and I didn't mind in the least. A bed was far more attractive than a singer and his guitar.

I stayed awake long enough to download and review one of my key medical records — the radiation plan, the plan that guided the beams from the machine that was zapping me Monday to Friday. Dr. Waldron had given me access to the hospital website holding the plan so I could make copies for myself and Dr. Norman back in St. John's.

This was really out of my league. It spoke of dose-grid geometry, photon beams and collimators. The Internet told me that the latter was a device to narrow a beam of radiation. The document was full of indecipherable abbreviations and medical gibberish from head to toe. But the pictures, now they were illuminating.

The radiation plan contained dozens of CT scans, every conceivable angle, from the top of my head to my shoulders. The plan designer had superimposed scores of contorted shapes on the slices, as they called them. Different colours for different dosages. My spinal cord had two shades of yellow traced along the full length. I assumed that was a low dosage zone. On other pictures there were blue, green, red, lavender, purple, lime and pink lines twisting every which way. It was as though a kid with an Etch-A-Sketch was in charge of the patterns.

The complexity was humbling. Dr. Waldron had told me that years ago a single plan could take days to write. Now, a computer did it in a couple of hours. The most striking image was of me in my immobilization mask. All colour was removed, and I looked like a mummy. The plan designer had traced the target zone on my face, neck and shoulders. My Adam's apple, the larynx, was outside the zone. The vocal cords were not receiving any radiation. Near my mouth, the line broke its pattern and jumped up, taking in the very spot where my left tonsil used to be. That area was getting the maximum radiation.

The oddest thing of all though, was the way the mask flattened my lips. It made them much bigger than usual. Maybe I did resemble a Maori wrasse after all.

Every November 11th as Canada remembers its war dead, I remember Corporal Jamie Murphy. He died January 27, 2004, when a suicide bomber threw himself at a jeep full of Canadian soldiers on patrol in Kabul, Afghanistan. Jamie Murphy was just twenty-six years old. And he will forever remind me that the longest walk a reporter ever takes is to a house with a grieving family inside.

Jamie Murphy grew up in Conception Harbour, Newfoundland. His parents' house is a forty-five-minute drive from St. John's. Just hours after Jamie was killed, I was knocking on their door.

Of all the things I do as a reporter, approaching a family in mourning is the one thing I dread. You can never predict the reception, and when it's hostile I feel terrible because I probably made the family's pain worse. But sometimes families want to talk and they've welcomed me. The "walk" has never gotten any easier over the years, nor should it.

Mr. Murphy's eyes were wet as he opened the door. He invited me in. I was so nervous that I forgot to introduce myself. I just started offering condolences and apologizing for intruding at a time when they were in so much anguish.

"Who are you?" one of the women asked.

"I'm Glenn Deir with CBC Television in St. John's," I sputtered.

They pulled out a chair at the kitchen table and we started chatting about Jamie. The room was full: Jamie's parents, two sisters, a brother-in-law, nephews and nieces, and neighbours. Out came the photographs, the Christmas postcard from Jamie, the tears. I found myself holding Mrs. Murphy's hand.

Their hearts were breaking and yet they found the strength to let a stranger into their home and treat him with the utmost courtesy and politeness. They understood why I was there.

"We want to honour Jamie," a sister said.

"Why don't you talk about this as a family? I'll wait outside in the van."

Cameraman Bruce Tilley and I discussed how we would handle the interview if it were granted. We would keep the lights to a minimum and not take the time to make the lighting perfect. This was no time to be fussy. If more than one person agreed to talk I would hold a single microphone, what we call a shotgun mic, a horrible name given the circumstances and one I would be careful not to use. A shotgun mic is tube-shaped and is excellent for picking up sound at a distance. That way we could all sit down comfortably and I wouldn't be in their faces.

After twenty minutes I knocked on the door again. Another polite welcome. The family had agreed to do an interview: Mr. and Mrs. Murphy and Jamie's sisters, Rosemary and Norma.

The four of them sat on a sofa in the living room beneath a photo of Jamie in camouflage fatigues. They had the eyes of people who have been crying for hours. They told me about the knock at five o'clock in the morning, with the priest and the military chaplain standing outside. They told me about their fears of Jamie going to Afghanistan, of his sense of duty and how he loved his job, of marking off the days on the calendar until Jamie's tour of duty ended, of the new house he had just bought with his girlfriend, and of the need to bring Canada's peace-keepers home from a place that doesn't want peace.

Mr. Murphy never said a word. At one point he couldn't take it anymore. He got up from the sofa and left the room. The three women immediately closed ranks. They sat closer together. Yes, there were tears, but not many. The women were thoughtful and articulate. If love alone could have protected him, Jamie Murphy would still be alive.

The interview was a journalistic coup and played across the country. I had emails from close friends; I had emails from people I never met. All of them offering congratulations and commending me for treating the family with dignity. I wondered whether I deserved the kind comments. I had put a distraught family on television in raw pain. It didn't seem very dignified.

On the day Jamie was buried, I was back in Conception Harbour for live inserts into our newscast. As the crew was breaking down the satellite truck, I went into the church hall. Jamie's sister, Rosemary, was still there. I shook her hand and told her again how sad I was for what happened. She didn't quite recognize me.

"You're the reporter who did the interview with us."

"Yes, I am. How was it?"

"I didn't see it, but I heard it was good."

Rosemary moved in and hugged me. This woman who bared her soul on television in her darkest hour hugged me. It meant more to me than all the accolades from my peers.

That's what I remember every November 11th. And fighting cancer didn't diminish the memory one iota.

"Stop ... asking ... me ... if ... I'm ... okay. I'm fine."

Deb had shown concern one time too many, and I snapped at her. She would freeze every time I had difficulty swallowing. A wince would make her eyes follow the spoon to my mouth, as if that bite might be my last.

"I'm feeling more like a hindrance than a supportive wife."

"I'm sorry. I'm not going to keel over and die. Please don't ask all the time if I'm okay."

I was irritable, and I needed more drugs. It was time to up the codeine dosage to the maximum allowable amount — 10 millilitres. I wondered if the extra codeine would turn my lower intestines into a pretzel again. Ever since my little "chat" with the nurse holding the rubber hose, I had been semi-regular, thanks to the chocolate-flavoured stool softener and cherry-flavoured laxative. I used to mix each with water or club soda, once in the morning and again before bedtime.

Sometimes, I'd stare at the glasses for a minute or two. My body really didn't want to be drinking those chocolate and cherry cocktails. I would feel the urge to throw up.

That urge came from other activities too. I would gag whenever I put a toothbrush towards the back of my mouth. Giving my molars a good cleaning was almost impossible.

My last few walks to Princess Margaret Hospital also caused my stomach to churn. It was as though my body knew that it was about to have more harm inflicted on it. I'd stop and close my eyes for a few seconds. The feeling would pass.

All in all, I felt like crap, and I was having a difficult time seeing the humour in it anymore.

"Damn."

I kept jabbing the blister on the inside lower lip with the

toothbrush bristles, which invariably caused a grimace and teeth sucking.

Deb couldn't do anything about that, but she certainly was trying to make me comfortable. I was really glad that she was there. The only thing worse than going through cancer treatment, is going through cancer treatment alone. However, I must admit that I wasn't showing enough gratitude or affection. I was being too Japanese for my own good.

One of my favourite stories on NHK World was something I called "Cabbage Patch Love." A crowd of Japanese men stood in a cabbage field yelling "I love you" to the women in their lives, to atone for all the times they hadn't said it. The report was hilarious. Japanese men are bashful, the story said, and are too shy to utter the words. I did a straw poll in the NHK newsroom. Ten out of ten women agreed.

"My father never said it to my mother."

"Only men in novels say it."

Tahira-san discreetly came by my desk and explained that a Japanese man who wishes to express his love would say something like, "The moon is particularly beautiful tonight." So, sometimes the moon is simply the moon and sometimes it's a metaphor for undying devotion.

I guess saying to Deb, "The CN Tower is particularly beautiful tonight" wasn't really cutting it.

Worse still, I went a little overboard playing the cancer card. Phrases like, "I've got cancer and you've got the comfortable chair" or "I've got cancer and I'd like the window open" were not all that endearing. By midweek, Deb was exasperated.

"I want the cancer gone by 9:30 Friday morning," she demanded. "I'm not taking it back to Newfoundland."

I guess I had it coming.

Even my curmudgeonly self could not help but smile at the Santa's Toyland display in the windows of the Hudson's Bay store.

Santa was standing in the balcony with a very long naughty and nice list, as the elves scrambled to get the toys ready. It was delightful. It reminded me of how exciting Christmas was when I was a kid, of the hours spent flipping through the Eaton's Christmas catalogue. Santa and his troupe didn't make me buy anything at The Bay, but they certainly gave me a glow.

Deb and I strolled along Queen Street. My cell phone rang. It was Steve, calling from the Gaff Topsails, our hunting grounds. The Gaff is a plateau in central Newfoundland, named after a gigantic knob of rock that resembles a gaff-topsail on a schooner. It's a wild and wonderful place. When my father was a boy, he and his parents were on a train that got stuck in a snowdrift there for three days. The rescuers had to dig them out.

The train and the tracks are all gone now. In previous Novembers, Steve and I had driven the old railway bed through trees and bogs in search of caribou. I had a hunting licence that fall, but returned it before flying to Toronto. Dr. Norman in St. John's had written a letter to wildlife officials, explaining that I couldn't hunt because of illness and treatment. The words "Radiation Oncologist" and "Cancer Care Program" were beneath her signature. Once again, there was no hiding my cancer, but it was the price I had to pay. By turning the licence back in, I would be eligible for another in the fall of 2008.

Steve and Jim, father-in-law to both of us, had just toasted the caribou they had killed. Old Sam black rum was in their glasses. I was happy for them, but a little sad for myself. Steve said it was the largest stag he had ever taken. There'd be plenty of caribou steaks, roasts and sausages in the freezer that winter.

I could picture exactly where they were. It was near the bog where I had shot a stag three years before. The Gaff Topsails is a place of personal contradiction. It's a land where I am at peace, and it's a land where I kill.

"I'll be there next year, Steve."

"So, it's almost Graduation Day," said Dr. Waldron. Graduation Day was the running joke around the lodge and hospital for those finishing radiation treatment. He glanced at the nurse's notes. She had weighed me before sending me into the examination room. I had dropped sixteen pounds in five weeks.

"A 10 per cent weight loss is acceptable." I was within acceptable limits.

"Dr. Waldron, I went through the radiation plan over the weekend. It was all Greek to me."

"Half of it is Greek to me too."

God, I thought, I hope he's kidding.

"I finally have your pathology results. You're HPV positive."

This was exciting news, at least to me. At my request, Dr. Waldron had sent my tissue samples off to Princess Margaret's pathology lab. I wanted to know if I was carrying the human papillomavirus. That might explain my cancer. Nothing else made sense. The other risk factors for throat cancer aren't a part of my life. I don't abuse alcohol, and I don't smoke. HPV is a leading suspect for my type of cancer and now I had the proof, not a smoking gun, but enough to issue an indictment. Sex probably gave me cancer.

Several studies show that people with cancerous tumours linked to HPV have significantly improved survival rates. HPV positive patients tend to respond better to radiation treatment. However, Dr. Waldron wasn't nearly as pleased as I was.

"Don't put too much stock in this."

Yes, this was a good thing, he explained, but the bigger and more beneficial factors were the small tumour in my tonsil and the small spot of cancer in the lymph node taken from my neck. Small was the key word.

"I'd rather be HPV negative with your tumour, than be HPV positive with a much bigger tumour."

Still, Dr. Waldron conceded that there is no sure way to predict a patient's outcome.

"I've had patients with small tumours who should have

survived and didn't, and I've had patients with large tumours who I thought wouldn't make it and they're still alive today."

It was time to move on. On top of my list of questions: how and when should I wean myself off the codeine?

That was really up to me, just don't do it in a day, he advised. Cut back gradually. One resident doctor predicted I'd probably be off the codeine within two weeks. I had trouble imagining it, given how vital the codeine was to my pain management.

"Dr. Waldron, this may seem like an odd question, and I only ask it because I've been to Hiroshima and Nagasaki, and have wondered about radiation sickness. What would have happened if you had given me all 60 gray at once?"

"I've been to Hiroshima, too. I tell people that I can kill every cancer cell in your body, absolutely, 100 per cent guaranteed. The problem is I'd kill 95 per cent of the healthy cells too."

He described what happens inside a human body exposed to lethal doses of radiation. It's utterly hideous — the lungs melt.

"A full body dose of just 4 gray would require a bone marrow transplant to save a life. We used 60 gray as a gamma knife. A very targeted strike to decimate a tumour."

High-energy radiation breaks up the DNA inside cancer cells and kills them. The healthy cells close by can usually recover, though my dead salivary glands are proof that there are limits. During an ordinary dental x-ray the jaw absorbs about .0025 gray. I was bombarded with 60 gray. No wonder I was fighting radiation sickness.

It was time to go. Dr. Waldron said the next time I was passing through Toronto, he'd like to see me. I thanked him for his care.

"I'll be watching for you on the telly," he said in a mock Newfoundland accent as he walked out the door.

He gave it a good try, but he was no Susumu. I thought, Worst Newfoundland accent since Julianne Moore in *The Shipping News*.

The sound of the cicada in Hiroshima was deafening. Before coming to Japan, I had never heard them. They "sing" best in the heat, and August 6, 2006, was scorching in Hiroshima. Just like it was sixty-one years before when the United States dropped Little Boy, and ushered the world into the horrors of nuclear warfare.

I was part of NHK's team broadcasting the memorial services in both Hiroshima and Nagasaki. It was an assignment I desperately wanted. I don't remember the first time I saw film of the mushroom cloud over Hiroshima, but the image has always been frighteningly seductive. Robert Oppenheimer said, "I am become death, the destroyer of worlds." I wanted to see what the father of the A-Bomb had wrought.

I walked over the T-shaped bridge that the bombardier of the *Enola Gay* used to locate his target. Little Boy exploded 600 metres overhead. I stood underneath the very spot. It was hard to believe that a fireball had obliterated every living thing there. What was once a burnt plain was now tropically lush. Hell was green.

The enduring symbol of August 6, 1945, is the Atomic Bomb Dome. The former exhibition hall was quite striking in its day. The distinctive feature was a centre tower with a copper dome. When the bomb exploded, much of the building was pummelled into rubble. But the tower miraculously survived. The dome was stripped clean; the copper vaporized. You can still look through the steel skeleton.

The human casualties of that day are graphically on display at Hiroshima's Peace Memorial Museum. I entered, wondering about the context. Japanese ultra-nationalists spin the story that the U.S. dropped the bomb while Japan was minding its own business.

The exhibits first laid out the pre-bomb history, such as the invasion of China. Japan fought a limited war in Manchuria in 1931, and then swept across the rest of China in 1937. To this day, China has not fully forgiven Japan.

The ultra-nationalists are not in charge at the Peace Memorial Museum. An exhibit sign said that Hiroshima's citizens celebrated Japan's military occupation of Nanking with a lantern parade but, "In Nanking, however, Chinese were being slaughtered by the Japanese Army." I felt relief. Relief, because in this museum at least, Japan's atrocities were acknowledged.

Compare that version of history to the one at Yasukuni Shrine in Tokyo. The shrine is home to the souls of Japan's war dead. When I was there, the shrine's museum vaguely spoke of the Nanking "incident." Nothing of the 300,000 civilians that China estimates were murdered, nothing of the thousands of women who were raped.

Thankfully, in Hiroshima there was candour. To me, it's an issue of credibility. It's hard to accept Japan's condemnation of nuclear bomb atrocities if it disavows the blood on its own hands.

The photos in the Peace Memorial Museum are ghastly. Flesh was incinerated, just like the copper on the A-Bomb Dome. The suffering must have been terrible. The most moving displays involve personal belongings: a lunch box with carbonized food, tattered school uniforms, and a tricycle that was once buried with a little boy in his parents' backyard.

Is an agonizing death from radiation more horrible than an agonizing death from a bayonet? Probably not. But Hiroshima gets the dubious honour of reminding us annually of the insanity of nuclear warfare. Every year, tens of thousands gather to pray for the souls of the dead. At 8:15 am, the exact moment of the explosion, everyone stands, and a single bell tolls throughout the Peace Park. The bell is struck by a battering ram of sorts. The sound is haunting.

During our broadcast, I was the voice of Prime Minister Junichiro Koizumi, the Mayor of Hiroshima, and two sixth graders. As they spoke Japanese, I read their speeches in English to the television audience. A colleague fluent in both languages gave me hand signals to keep me on track. The kids gave the best speech.

We ask, "What is peace?" Peace is without strife or wars.
It is without bullying or violence, without crimes, poverty
or hunger.

Peace is being able to go to school in safety. It's studying, playing and eating.
Being able to live one day just like any other day is also peace.

They understood what happened to their grandparents and vowed to prevent it from happening again.

That evening, Deb and I joined my NHK friends for grilled meat on skewers and cabbage with soy sauce. The beer never stopped flowing and neither did the chorus of "Kampai!" *Cheers!*

We talked about the Peace Memorial Museum. My Japanese colleagues felt the history was balanced. The A-Bomb is not a topic I had broached with them before. I had been squeamish about it because the sins of the father are not the sins of the son. Even though some Japanese whitewash their country's war crimes, Japan has not gone to war since 1945. War is outlawed in their constitution. Japan also pledges not to make nuclear bombs, or possess them, or allow them into the country. The hawk has become a dove.

With the Hiroshima memorial service over, we caught the bullet train to Nagasaki. Human nature attaches lesser status to those in second place. That holds true even for atomic bombs. The Nagasaki Atomic Bomb Museum is not as prestigious as Hiroshima's, but it's no less compelling. They have a photo that says more about the bomb than all the words ever written. It's a silhouette of a man and a ladder. The bomb vaporized both the man and the ladder, but their images stayed on a clapboard wall. They blocked the searing heat, allowing it to change the colour of the wall around their shadows.

The memorial ceremony in Nagasaki was a much more intimate affair. Our broadcast booth was only ten metres from Prime Minister Koizumi's seat. I knew he was popular, but I didn't realize he had rock star appeal. His entrance sent a buzz through the school children. They were up on their feet, and their faces showed that they were thrilled. The PM waved a couple of times to acknowledge the adoration. Meanwhile, his massive security detail scanned the crowd. One officer was carrying an overcoat in broiling heat. I suspected he was hiding something lethal underneath it.

Koizumi's speech was a carbon copy of the one he gave three days before. He merely replaced the word Hiroshima with Nagasaki. He romped through the speech, so fast in fact, that I was still speaking as he walked away from the podium. The prime minister offered no emotion, no originality. My Japanese colleagues explained that he probably did this to show no favouritism.

I was also the voice of a woman who spoke about her memories of August 9, 1945. The Japanese created a word to describe people like Kikuyo Nakamura; she is a hibakusha — an atomic blast survivor. Her speech was all the things that Koizumi's was not.

> *Voices around me told me not to give the wounded water, but I soaked up water with a towel and wrung it into their mouths. "Thank you," they said in a very thin voice, and smiling faintly, died. People were crying "Mother!" with their last breath and I was forced to watch helplessly as the young people around me died one by one.*
>
> *Only three years ago my second son became a victim of the bombing, dying from leukemia at fifty-five years of age, despite not even being alive the day the bomb was dropped. Instead he was doomed by the lingering radiation. I shall never forget what the doctor said to me: "You passed the cause of the leukemia to your son Hiroshi." Those words torment me to this day.*

Friday, November 16, 2007, was "Graduation Day." It did not start auspiciously. I woke up with nausea. Breakfast was my usual soft-boiled egg and a cocktail of milk and Boost. It took me thirty minutes to get them down, and once I returned to the room, only three seconds to bring them up. I retched several times over the toilet, and barely had the strength to make it back to the bed. I could only allow myself a few minutes' rest. My appointment was for 8:35, and I was going to make it, even if I had to crawl to Princess Margaret Hospital.

Deb and I walked past Maple Leaf Gardens. The fresh air revived me. We bumped into another lodge resident on his way to radiation treatment too. Doctors had discovered cancer in the roof of his mouth. They cut it out and reconstructed the bone. He joked with his friends, "I'm going off to the spa for a week." Obviously, I didn't have a monopoly on black humour.

The "convocation" could not have been more routine. Instead of an academic gown, I was offered a johnny coat. I declined, just as I had on twenty-four previous occasions. I still preferred to be bare-chested. It was cooler and more comfortable.

"What's your date of birth?" One final safety check.

"January 22, 1958."

The whirls, clicks, grinding and growling from the radiation machine went through their usual refrain.

"All done for the last time," said one of the radiation therapists as they released the mask bolting me to the table. They remarked on how little skin damage they had caused. The Evil Glenn wondered if that was a note of approval, or disappointment. By damage, they were referring to seeping cracks in my skin. I also had two dozen tiny scabs around my neck. Apparently, that was getting off easy. I was lobster-red from my chin to my collarbones. It was the kind of appearance that would prompt the sea captain on *The Simpsons* to mutter, "'Tis neither man nor beast."

The lobster-red was everywhere except my Adam's apple. That area had its normal skin colour and texture, and my beard was still growing there. It was as though someone had laid a silver dollar on the spot during all treatments, protecting my larynx from the x-rays. The healthy skin brilliantly showed the flexibility of the IMRT treatment. Despite damage all around it, my voice box was unhurt. Now, if only I could get the marbles out of my mouth, I might be a television reporter again some day.

I didn't get a degree on my Graduation Day, just a warm handshake from the radiation therapist and a "Good luck." He went to wipe my name from the board and someone had already done it. The corpse wasn't even cold and the mourning was already over. Radiation treatment is a volume business and space is at a premium. Move along please is the underlying sentiment.

As I was leaving the radiation unit, I bumped into a couple from Manitoba whom I'd met at the lodge. Her radiation would end in a couple of days. We shook hands and wished each other well. We each chose safe words. I had no idea about her prognosis, nor she mine. Neither of us was making assumptions.

Five weeks, twenty-five treatments. I was finished. The millstone had turned into a milestone. While Princess Margaret Hospital didn't give me an academic title, I didn't walk away empty-handed. I took the immobilization mask. I didn't want it, me — the Ghostly Glenn — tossed in the dumpster, at least not yet. As I was leaving the hospital a woman stopped me.

"Excuse me, but would you please tell me what that is?"

"A better question might be, 'Who is that?'"

"That's you," she exclaimed, delighted with her own deduction.

I explained what the mask was and how it was used. I wasn't sure what I'd do with it back home. Perhaps terrorize the neighbourhood kids next Halloween. I doubted that it would replace the David Blackwood print over the fireplace.

What should have been a day of celebration was tarnished by a conversation I overheard in the lodge's elevator. One of the bald beauties started chatting with a guy with a suitcase.

"Going home?"

"Yes, it's been a long five weeks."

I cringed. I had learned that five weeks in the lodge didn't begin to qualify as long.

"I've been here five months," she said, "and I just found out that I have to go back into hospital next week. The stem cell transplant didn't take."

"I'm sure it will next time," he said, as he wheeled his suitcase off the elevator.

No doubt his five weeks were no fun, but I had a hard time feeling any empathy. He had no business being cavalier to that woman.

Victories came in all shapes and sizes at the lodge. Take Pete from northern Ontario. His stem cell transplant did work, and a few days earlier he was given permission to spend more time with his new grandson. After four months of exile in Toronto, he could finally pack his suitcase and go home. He was walking on air. I was happy for him. People seemed happy for me too when they learned that I was leaving. There was good will enough for all, and it was freely offered to everyone. Apart from Mr. It's-Been-A-Long-Five-Weeks, no one seemed to think that he or she was entitled to it.

"Are you going to be all right?" asked Deb.

The swaying of the taxi ride to the airport was getting the better of me. I wasn't sure that I could keep my stomach down. I was never so happy to see a departures ramp.

Deb and I rested on seats near a washroom. I bolted. I never made it to a toilet stall. A washroom sink was as far as I got. I threw up several times. Black and green phlegm. Fortunately, no one else was around. I cleaned the sink, washed my face and shuffled back to Deb.

"Get ... me ... through ... security ... now."

"Why?"

I didn't answer. Deb looked at my ashen face and said, "Right."

I passed out on the plane. I remember taking off in Toronto and landing in St. John's, nothing in between.

We walked in through the front door around midnight. I dropped the Ghostly Glenn in the hallway and headed upstairs to get ready for bed. I was home.

Poster Boy

I'm going to take a moment to apologize to Dr. Boyd Lee, Dr. Alia Norman, Dr. John Waldron and Dr. Michael Kennedy, my family doctor. Dr. Kennedy's only "crime" was being a stellar GP and pouncing on the bulge in my neck, thereby setting off the chain of events that led to this moment. I apologize not for something I've said, but for something I'm about to say. My apology is without qualification or reservation, and is absolutely necessary. My comments will be ill-considered, impolite, vulgar, disrespectful, boorish, ungracious, unwarranted and offensive.

As I've mentioned previously, radiation has a cumulative effect. It hit its peak in those first few days at home. My body was in open rebellion because of radiation sickness. I fluctuated between collapsing into the bed from exhaustion and running to the bathroom to throw up. One morning was particularly vile. There was nothing left in my stomach, and yet I continued to retch over the toilet. I wiped a little spittle off my mouth and sat back. I was afraid to leave. Good thing too. I vomited again.

As I lifted my head out of the toilet bowl, I imagined all the doctors who had cared for me.

"You BASTARDS did this to me. Cancer never made me puke until I got the dry heaves. Cancer never burned and cracked my skin. Cancer never killed my salivary glands. Cancer never stole my energy. Cancer never made my mouth hurt. Cancer never made me stop running. Cancer never made me feel god-awful. Cancer never did a damn thing to me. You BASTARDS did this to me."

I felt wonderful before the doctors began "curing" me. Of course, these very same doctors might have saved my life by making me so sick. Without their intervention, there was a good chance I would have faced a horrific future. On that morning though, I couldn't see it. I was full of bile. Please refer back to my apology in the first paragraph.

"Nan and Leet have a soft spot for you," said Deb.

"I don't know why," I said.

"Neither do I."

Deb had just told me that her Grandmother Churchill and Aunt Valeda were including me in their nightly prayers. Leet, as everyone in the family calls her, was showing incredible generosity because she was fighting ovarian cancer herself. Leet had also arranged for my name to be read aloud every Sunday during the sick and healing prayers at the Anglican Church in nearby Portugal Cove. I wasn't raised an Anglican, and I had never set foot inside that church, and yet people who didn't personally know me were asking God to make me well.

The prayer campaign didn't end there. Mary Jane's mom in Dartmouth was praying for me, Sue in Bermuda was praying for me, and Deb's Grandmother Youden in Topsail was praying for me. It was all very humbling.

However, I also felt unworthy. Frankly, I'm not that nice of a person. A nice person wouldn't use, as Mom would say, a bad word to describe his doctors. A nice person wouldn't snap at his concerned wife. There had to be other people who deserved divine intervention more than I did. I hadn't bothered to pray at all. Not a single prayer from the moment I was diagnosed with cancer.

Even though I was raised in a United Church home and attended services regularly until my mid-teens, I am a non-believer.

I can point to no single cause or event. I've never had a crisis of faith, because I've never had faith. So, I felt a tad embarrassed that people would mention my name to a benevolent deity whose existence I doubted. I never asked people to stop though. Prayer could do no harm and for all I knew, it might have been doing a great deal of good.

My lack of faith didn't stop me from carrying a god in Tokyo. Several times in one day, in fact. It happened during the Sanja Festival in Asakusa, home to one of Tokyo's best-known temples. Once a year, the three gods who inhabit the temple are carried through the streets of Asakusa in portable shrines called mikoshi.

I fell into the opportunity through sheer luck. A friend knew a friend whose dad was organizing a team for the mikoshi parade and they needed people with strong backs. A mikoshi resembles a miniature temple. They are quite ornate; the one I helped carry had a gold peacock perched on top. The mikoshi sits on four 4 by 4 beams, and it takes about three dozen people to lift it.

One has to dress the part to be a mikoshi bearer. I was given a happi coat — a light cotton jacket, fastened with a belt. The district's emblem was on the back. On my feet were brilliant white tabi boots. They had a split-toe look, meaning the big toe was separated from the other toes. Protecting my head from the blistering sun was a bandana stamped "Intel Inside," a reference not to my computing power but our corporate sponsor. Being a gaijin, I was a star attraction. The camera clicks never stopped. Complete strangers were yelling, "Smile."

Carrying a mikoshi is a lot like riding a horse. If you don't find the right rhythm, a part of you will get very sore, very quickly. The mikoshi sat on our shoulders. It was unwieldy and had a mind of its own. Sometimes, it was one step forward, two steps back. The mikoshi was heaving up and down, staggering all over the place like the town drunk.

Mikoshi bearers spoon. It's a practical matter. That kind of intimate togetherness is the only way to get enough carriers underneath the mikoshi to lift it. Being taller than the others, I was using a semi-squat walk. It took only minutes for my shoulders and thighs to ache. The secret to survival was rotating in and out of the group, and switching shoulders. Otherwise, I would have acquired welts the size of grapefruits. There was drumming, and there were chants of "Soi-ya, soi-ya" as we made our way through the throngs. It was exhilarating. After twenty minutes, we passed the mikoshi to the next group.

At the time, I hoped that the god appreciated the effort. Perhaps I survived cancer because he did.

Steve was a terrific morale booster in those early days back in St. John's. He and I walked around Long Pond daily, though preparing for the walk took almost as much time as the walk itself. I had a terrible "sunburn" on my neck and shoulder blades. The skin was blistered, cracked and moist in spots, though it looked far worse than it felt. Still, my skin needed protection from the chafing of a heavy sweater and coat.

Step one was cleaning the skin, which encouraged quite a bit of stinging because I was using a homemade saline solution. Who the hell thought it would be a good idea to direct patients to pour salt water on open wounds? I soaked a facecloth in the solution and laid it on my burned skin for ten minutes, gently wiping away any of the dead bits afterwards.

I then smeared the entire area with a sticky ointment designed to form a protective barrier over severely damaged skin. I laid sterile pads on the ointment and wrapped gauze right around the whole kit and caboodle. Steve often helped attach the gauze to my upper chest and back with surgical tape. Thank God, the radiation had stripped away my body hair. It took thirty minutes of prep work before I could take a step outside.

I was chilled to the bone, no matter how many layers I wore. I scrunched my coat and scarf together in a futile attempt to keep the cold wind out. I shivered my way around Long Pond, and I always seemed short of breath. I needed the fresh air and exercise though, so staying inside wasn't a serious option. Only the vilest of weather cancelled a walk.

By the fall of 2007, mothers and fathers throughout Newfoundland and Labrador would have been thinking a great deal about their young daughters' health. The province began vaccinating grade six girls against the human papillomavirus. The vaccine protects girls against four types of HPV, the types that account for most cervical cancers and genital warts. The idea is to immunize girls before they become sexually active.

My mind was reeling at the poster boy possibilities. I could see my face on billboards along major highways, with foot-high letters.

What Does This Galoot of a Man Have in Common With Your Eleven-Year-Old Daughter? More Than You Think!

That would certainly get the attention of shotgun-toting fathers everywhere. But I'm not interested in getting shot. I have a message for dads and moms, and it's not about their daughters. It's about their sons.

By the fall of 2007, I knew I was HPV positive. I also knew that HPV infection is strongly associated with throat cancer. What caused my poster boy flight of fancy was stumbling across an article in the *New England Journal of Medicine*. It told me that I could have been carrying the HPV virus for a decade or more, that I probably picked it up during oral sex, that the rates of tonsil and tongue cancer are on the rise, and that there is a strong case for vaccinating little boys against HPV, as well as little girls.

I had an epiphany: Glenn Deir, coming to a poster near you.

As a child, I was vaccinated against tuberculosis. The twenty-first century has a new scourge that school kids should be protected against. Little boys will grow up and they will have sex.

Without protection, they risk contracting HPV. You don't want your little boy going through what I went through.

"It will take time to get back to where I was," I said to Deb over breakfast.

"I was kind of hoping that you would go beyond that," she replied.

Same contempt that I saw in the cancer clinic months before. Deb must have thought that I was getting better.

I certainly didn't feel it. Not to put too fine a point on it, but the first two weeks after my radiation treatment ended were hellish. I was constantly fighting nausea, coughing up disgusting amounts of phlegm, and bowel movements were torturous.

It was during week three that I scowled at the bottles of stool softener and laxative. "I can't drink any more of this crap." But I had to wean myself off the codeine first. I decreased my dosage to half, and after several days, I went cold turkey. There was no screaming pain.

Around the same time, I opened a bottle of Boost and my stomach rolled over. "I can't drink any more of this crap." I started eating soft food again. A couple of days later, I dropped the Boost altogether. Pureed soups and peanut butter on moist bagels soon became staples. Best of all, the peanut butter tasted like peanut butter. My taste buds had survived.

I looked like I had just been released from a Serbian POW camp. I was gaunt. No surprise really when I stepped on the scales at the cancer clinic that December morning. The two-week liquid diet and stomach evacuation exercises had caused my weight to plummet. I had dropped twenty-four pounds since starting radiation. Even though I was back on soft food, Doctors Lee and Norman were definitely going to be seeing a much thinner Glenn Deir.

"Your beard is gone," said Dr. Norman, seemingly struck

more by my baby faced appearance than my emaciated physique. The radiation whacked my beard like a Soprano hit. Shaving was history, except for a small patch over my voice box and a thin line below each cheekbone. The very action that led to the discovery of the lump in my neck in the first place was no longer an integral part of my daily routine.

The doctors seemed very happy with the way I looked, but I didn't share their enthusiasm and was full of complaints. My tongue was swollen, my cheeks were puffy, the skin around my neck was starting to peel, and I had an ugly zit on my chin. And that was only part of the list.

"Don't pop the zit," said Dr. Lee. He explained that it was caused by radiation and would eventually disappear.

"I wake up every morning coughing up black phlegm. Is that because the inside of my throat was burned like the outside?" Both doctors nodded.

I was talking through clenched teeth, and it was obvious to Dr. Norman.

"How many fingers can you get in your mouth?"

I gingerly opened my mouth and slipped in my index and middle fingers. I winced. My jaw joints had radiation-induced stiffness.

"How many can you get in *your* mouth?"

"This many." She pushed in three fingers. "I want you to do mouth stretching exercises. Two or three fingers in the mouth, hold one minute, three times a day."

Dr. Lee wanted a look inside. I opened my mouth as best I could, but it hurt. Parts of my throat and tongue were still inflamed. The worst area was where my left tonsil used to be. Both doctors said not to think about returning to work until I was eating normally and my throat and tongue were better.

"Don't brush your tongue or the roof of your mouth when you're brushing your teeth," said Dr. Lee.

"No alcohol over Christmas," said Dr. Norman. "Just a little champagne New Year's Eve. Alcohol slows down the healing."

"Food is a chore. I have no appetite. I eat because I must, but I don't enjoy it. If I didn't look at the clock, I wouldn't know that it's lunch time."

"I know," said Dr. Lee. "You're a textbook case. It's perfectly normal. Your appetite will come back."

Textbook case. I was Mr. Dull as a patient, about as far away from Glenn-san Syndrome as one could possibly get. The Evil Glenn imagined Dr. Lee entertaining other doctors at the staff Christmas party with the story of how this Deir guy was sooooo ordinary, but he had delusions of having a disease named after him. That should get a few laughs.

"You know, the question everyone keeps asking me is, 'Why didn't they take both tonsils?'"

Dr. Lee repeated what I already knew. If he had done the surgery instead of Dr. Burrage, he would have taken both. Dr. Burrage had a different point of view.

"But we found the primary source," said Dr. Lee. He explained that the tonsils operate as different entities, and it wasn't likely that the cancer would travel to the right tonsil.

"Are you using your dental trays?" asked Dr. Norman.

I confessed no, and gave her my tale of woe about the burning fluoride gel. She didn't seem impressed and strongly encouraged me to pop them back in.

"They've been proven effective."

I knew she was right. I'd have to start wearing them again and the sooner the better. The survival of my teeth depended on it. I took a couple of sips from my water bottle, my ever-present companion.

"Dr. Lee, how will I ever run again with a dry mouth?"

He looked completely baffled. "I have no idea. No one has ever asked me that question before. Most of my patients are two-pack-a-day smokers or 40-ouncer-a-day drinkers. They don't ask me about jogging."

I was constantly sipping while not running. How would I manage when I started trotting again? I owned a water bottle and holster for jogging, but I couldn't take the bottle out every minute or two.

Dr. Lee told me about a drug he could prescribe to encourage my salivary glands to secrete more, but it had potentially unpleasant side effects. The saliva could be thick, and I might sweat profusely. The medical solution was not very appealing.

"Oh, before I forget, Cynthia says 'Hello,'" I said.

You know you live in a small city when the woman who cuts your hair knows the man who removed a cancerous lump off your jugular vein. When Cynthia first saw the scar on my neck and heard the name Boyd Lee, she casually mentioned that they knew each other in high school.

Dr. Lee transformed instantly. He went from a guy with mussed-up hair to a hunk doctor from the TV show *ER*.

"She was my first girlfriend, I think. It's hard to remember, there were so many."

The medical student in the back was clearly impressed. "It's all coming out now," she said.

Dr. Lee doesn't look like George Clooney, not in the least, but was I going to argue with a man who stuck a scalpel in my neck? No. Shutting up seemed like the smart thing to do.

On the way home, Deb jokingly suggested the solution to my jogging problem was one of those ball caps that can hold two beer — the sort of cap worn by pot-bellied guys in T-shirts at race-tracks. Each beer has a hose for sipping. I laughed, but Deb was on to something. I'd have to check out water packs with hoses.

It was a tough day all round, despite the doctors glowing assessment. I was battling the Sleep Demon, diarrhea, nausea, coughing and phlegm. I just wanted to feel better and was sick of being sick.

I'm constantly failing the three wise monkeys. I have no choice; it's in my nature and besides, if I didn't see evil, hear evil and speak evil, journalism would have nothing to do with me. I'd be out of a job.

That bluntness gets me in trouble sometimes, but it also got me to Japan to see the sage threesome. A carving of them, perhaps *the* carving of them, is at a shrine in Nikko. The shrine also houses the tomb of the shogun Ieyasu Tokugawa. He was Japan's great unifier, ending centuries of feudal wars. He did it mostly by being a conniving, murderous dictator, who even executed his first wife and eldest son because it was politically advantageous to do so.

Those wooden primates were probably a warning to everyone around the Tokugawa clan: if you want to see sunrise, you had better keep your eyes covered, your ears plugged, and your mouth shut. Words to live by. Alas, I can never seem to follow good advice.

Now that I was home, perhaps Okawa-san suspected I needed tempering. He sent me a note with a wonderful sentiment.

There is an old Japanese saying, now that you got a disease you should make it a friend so that you will be able to live long.

Okawa-san was right, as always. There was no point in hating cancer. There was no point in railing against my doctors. The time for anger was over. I was going to have to make peace with my cancer and my cure. See no evil, hear no evil, and speak no evil.

I should have told my doctors in my best John Cleese impersonation, "You turned me into a Newt."

In the movie, *Monty Python and the Holy Grail,* a peasant accuses a woman of being a witch because she turned him into a newt. The peasant is referring to a salamander. I'm referring to a teacher named Newt.

Deb made the mistake of describing my speech impediment and clenched teeth to her sister Linda. Did I get sympathy? No. Did I get pity? No. I was mocked instead.

Linda was practically giddy when she wrote. She once had a high school teacher named Newton. He was a frail, elderly man with a crewcut who spoke through clenched teeth. That's who I reminded her of.

How many more indignities would I have to endure? I was a Newt.

I couldn't spend the rest of my life as a Newt, and Dr. Norman's mouth exercises didn't seem to be working, so I saw a physiotherapist. She recommended an exercise she called guppy mouth. I opened my mouth as wide as I could, while keeping my tongue pressed behind my upper teeth. Repeat ten times, six times a day. I was so faithful to the regime that I absent-mindedly found myself doing guppy mouth while driving down a main road in St. John's. I can't imagine what the oncoming drivers were thinking. Maybe it was the exercise, maybe it was natural healing, or maybe it was a combination of both, but within a couple of weeks I was no longer a Newt.

I excitedly said to Deb, "I can put two knuckles in my mouth now with no pain."

"That's great. Can I put a fist in?"

"I'm going to pray for you," said Anna.

I was floored. Deb and I had only met Anna and her husband that evening. We were all dinner guests. A month had passed since my return from Toronto, and this was my coming-out party. We spent a portion of it reliving the Bruce Springsteen concert because they had been there too. My health was naturally the subject of a few questions, and I thought nothing more of it until Anna held my hand and made her promise. This was no casual commitment; her eyes told me this was a vow. I felt so unworthy and embarrassed again.

By Christmas Day I was eating just about everything that New-foundlanders grow, catch or kill, which is a frighteningly long list. Santa had filled my stocking with optimism. Hot mustard, spicy coriander sauce and a Tuborg beer, which was brewed especially for Christmas. All were still off limits. Someday my taste buds would delight in them, but not Christmas Day.

Bland was beautiful. Nothing spicy, nothing acidic. No orange juice, no tomato, no curry. Despite my limitations, I was enjoying food again. I still wasn't feeling hunger pangs, but when I told my body that it was time to eat I could savour the taste. Salmon with dill, lamb with rosemary, Christmas turkey with mashed turnip and butter. I was so thankful that I had defied the worst-case scenario in the medical literature.

Deb and I celebrated New Year's Eve at Karen and Steve's. After countless glasses of club soda, I was ready to try a bubbly drink containing alcohol. I had my eye on the chilled 1996 Pol Roger champagne. Steve suddenly waved a bottle of cheap sparkling wine around.

"Here, give Deir that. He can't taste the difference."

We all laughed, but Steve's joke was probably true. However, I'd be damned if I was going to pass up a glass of quality champagne. The bubbles danced on my tongue, but there was slight burning too. I wasn't ready for very much alcohol.

We dined on grilled shrimp, Coquille Saint Jacques and pork tenderloin with a mixed berry sauce. Another classic meal from Chef Steve. Everything tasted as I remembered, however, there was no real way to know absolutely. I suspected my taste range had become narrower, but I couldn't prove my theory without before and after taste buds.

In the end, what did it matter? The best part of the meal wasn't the taste anyway. The best part was that it didn't have vanilla or strawberry flavour, it wasn't liquid, and it didn't come out of a plastic bottle.

Feeling Genki

Genki is one of my favourite Japanese words. It means energetic or healthy. I like the sound of it. It's crisp and punchy. I feel genki! I use it when I'm feeling great.

I was feeling genki enough in the early days of 2008 to spend an afternoon snowshoeing and then another cross-country skiing. The exertion and fresh air knocked me out early each evening. Still, they were proof that I was on the mend.

As the weeks rolled on, I ran out of patience. All the medical literature suggested that I could expect to lose the inflammation in my throat six to eight weeks after finishing radiation treatment. I woke up one Friday morning, eight weeks to the day after I graduated from the radiation program, and ordered my throat to get better instantly. My throat contemptuously ignored me, permitting acidic and spicy foods to sting all the more.

It wasn't supposed to be that way. Long before my treatment started, I had big plans for my birthday. On January 22, 2008, I was supposed to be in New York scaling the Empire State Building, seeing a Broadway show, and salivating over a street vendor pretzel. But noooo, that was too much to ask for.

I turned fifty in St. John's, not salivating over very much, I'm afraid, a lingering consequence of the radiation. Nonetheless, Deb arranged a unique meal for my half-century birthday dinner.

We ate horse, whale and puffin; the horse came from Quebec, while the latter two were imported from Iceland.

The puffin was particularly good. And no, it didn't taste like chicken. It had a saltwater duck flavour. The Evil Glenn thought, *It's a good thing Newfoundlanders don't know about this, or those protected puffin colonies in Witless Bay would be stripped naked.*

I first ate whale meat in Japan during an after-work soiree at a soba noodle restaurant. The menu was entirely in Japanese, but I flipped through it anyway, always looking to practice my Nihongo.

"What is kujira?" I asked in lurching Japanese.

"Whale!" said one of my NHK colleagues. "Want to try some?"

Perhaps they were playing let's gross out the gaijin, but they really picked the wrong guy for that. My stomach was built of steel. However, I hesitated saying yes. Maybe I had been on a whaleboat tour once too often. Maybe deep down I had succumbed to the idea that whales are too beautiful to kill. Maybe I was afraid that whales were endangered.

Japan calls its whale hunt "scientific research," thereby using a loophole to get around the international ban on whaling. I had a feeling that the scientific research was bogus, that it was commercial whaling by another name, and that its real purpose was to supply restaurants and grocery stores with delicious meat. The deceit bothered me. The Japanese fleet was gearing up to kill about one thousand minke and ten fin whales in the Antarctic. And the Japanese intended to do it proudly, despite withering condemnation from conservation groups and reservations from international scientists. Japan's own scientists said a hunt was sustainable.

What to do? The word hypocrite bounced around my brain. After all, I come from a place where fishermen kill cute seals, hundreds of thousands of them every year, eliciting diatribes from every corner of Christendom. The same environmentalists who heap scorn on Japanese heap scorn on Newfoundlanders, but the vitriolic abuse hasn't stopped me from eating seal a couple of times a year.

I was also mindful of the fact that I am a hunter. At that point, I had taken two caribou from the Gaff Topsails. There is nothing more majestic than a caribou stag bounding across a bog, and yet I was able to pull the trigger, twice.

I asked myself if I could stand on the same moral ground as Greenpeace, the Sea Shepherd Conservation Society and the International Fund for Animal Welfare. No, I couldn't. That thought was tougher to swallow than any piece of whale.

"Want to try some?"

"Yes."

The whale came raw and thinly sliced on a platter — elegantly presented, as sashimi always is in Tokyo. Whale is a dark red meat. The taste was subtle, the texture tender; it was quite succulent. I took only the one piece. Based on how quickly the rest of the whale disappeared, I was the only person at the table whose conscience was troubled.

"Jesus, what the hell is that?"

I couldn't believe what I was seeing. I ran and got a flashlight, shone it into my mouth and looked again in the bathroom mirror. I was horrified. There was black fuzz over much of my tongue, and even a few curly hairs on the very back. No one had warned me about this, whatever this was. I dashed to the computer and googled: black, tongue, radiation.

Apparently, I had a condition with the delightful name Black Hairy Tongue. The web pages screamed out, "POOR ORAL HYGIENE." I screamed back, "IT'S NOT MY FAULT. THE DOCTORS MADE ME."

I had been told not to brush my tongue when cleaning my teeth. The doctors didn't want me brushing away delicate tissue as I healed. That was fine as long as I was belting back my Cherry Kool-Aid mouthwash before every meal. It was one-third anti-fungal drug, so it kept such gothic coats at bay. However, I had given up the mouthwash by late January. While I still had a particularly sensitive spot on the side of my tongue, I no longer needed to numb my entire mouth and throat before eating. Since I was off the Kool-Aid and my tongue wasn't getting its usual sloughing, tiny bumps on the surface grew like weeds and bacteria ran amok.

I was relieved to discover that my tongue wasn't going to fall out and the black fuzz wasn't cancer. The cure was simple: brush my tongue. I started with light brushings, ever mindful that I wasn't completely healed. The medical web sites promised that my tongue would return to its normal appearance within a few weeks.

If Mick Jagger had ever suffered through an episode of Black Hairy Tongue, I doubt he would have chosen a tongue logo for The Rolling Stones.

I was a little rash in dubbing myself Baby Face Glenn. My moustache started growing again, as did my sideburns and the beard on my cheeks. My neck, however, stayed as smooth as a baby's bottom. All of which was a pain in the ass, frankly. A blotchy beard would not do. I was using a borrowed electric razor, had been since I started radiation treatment. Razor blades were considered too sharp for my delicate skin. Electric razors give a lousy shave, but I would have to wait until my skin was completely healed before returning to shaving foam, twin blades and long strokes.

Still, I was presentable when I saw Cynthia to get my hair cut. She discovered a problem as she fussed about. The hairline on the back of my neck was higher than it used to be. I hadn't thought of that radiation side effect since Dr. Waldron mentioned it months before. I explained that the radiation went in through the front and came out on the back of the neck, killing hair cells along the way. Cynthia and I chatted about my time in Toronto as she shaped my curly hair to cover-up the bare spot.

"Will it ever come back?" she asked.

"The doctors say I have a 90 per cent chance of a cure."

"I have some other clients and it came back."

"Really." My heart sank. Yet another reminder that the sword of Damocles was hanging over my head by a thread and it could still fall.

"Ya, fuller than ever," said Cynthia.

It was then that I realized she was talking about hair and I was talking about cancer. Cross purposes and misunderstandings. This is how train wrecks happen.

Time for a little teasing about the juicy bit I picked up at the cancer clinic. "You didn't tell me that you *dated* Boyd Lee."

Now that the secret was out, Cynthia confessed that she was the wild one; Dr. Lee was the studious type. She was the kind of girl who jumped out of the bedroom window when her parents grounded her and wouldn't let her go to the dance.

Imagine! That's the kind of company my neck surgeon once kept. And to think that I trusted my life with that man.

"Dr. Internet tells me that I have Black Hairy Tongue, but I wouldn't mind hearing what you've got to say," I said to Dr. Lee.

"Dr. Internet, eh." Dr. Lee was smiling. I was at the cancer clinic for a routine check-up. One was scheduled every two months. Dr. Lee looked in my mouth.

"Yes, that's what you've got."

The resident doctor, who was hanging on his every word, had no idea what we were talking about. He had never heard of such a thing before.

"Now you're scaring me," I said.

"Come on," said Dr. Lee, looking a little annoyed that I was giving his protégé a hard time.

"Is it caused by radiation?" the resident asked.

"No, not exactly," replied Dr. Deir.

Dr. Lee finally let him off the hook by filling in the blanks with medical gobbledygook. I was feeling quite smug. It's not every day that I upstage and torment a medical student. He got his revenge though. Dr. Lee invited him to push a rubber scope up my nose and down my throat.

"Breathe, please."

Taking in air opened up the nasal passage. I'll give the resident credit. He did a fine job with no anaesthetic spray. He looked through the scope and found that I still had swelling in my throat.

The doctors were seeing me at my best because it was early morning. I usually regressed as the day went along. There were times when my voice was scratchy and tired. Occasionally, I sounded like I was recovering from a cold, even though I was sniffle- and sneeze-free. Most annoying though, was not being able to form words properly. It was as though my tongue was too big for my mouth. Had I been on television, people would have been tuning in to see just how badly I could mangle the Queen's English. Nevertheless, returning to work was exactly what I had on my mind. Coincidently, Dr. Norman was thinking the same thing. Her motivation was encouraging a return to normal life. My motivation was money.

Shakespeare wrote: "The first thing we do, let's kill all the lawyers." I'd like to add: "and insurance case managers."

The day before, I had received a letter from Elizabeth R., case manager with the Great-West Life Insurance Company. My application for Long Term Disability benefits had been denied, on the grounds that I had consulted doctors (Dr. King in Tokyo and Dr. Kennedy in St. John's) about the lump in my neck and "received medical treatment" before returning to the Canadian Broadcasting Corporation and the protection of its insurance coverage.

I was facing a financial crisis. I had exhausted my sick leave and I was burning up my annual leave at a furious rate. I needed the insurance company to bridge the gap between the end of my annual leave and my return to work. Their rejection of my claim meant I would soon have no income whatsoever.

Great-West Life's decision was infuriating. In my view, seeing a doctor about a lump in my neck, asking advice and undergoing a physical exam did not constitute medical treatment. Prior to the report from the Armed Forces Institute of Pathology, there were only theories, conjecture and best guesses about my lump. My radiation treatment didn't start until well beyond the eligibility date for LTD benefits.

Perhaps most galling of all was the fact that someone named Elizabeth R. had signed the rejection letter. Elizabeth and her colleagues knew every intimate detail about my case. Dr. Waldron told them that I had throat cancer, that I received radiation therapy every day for five weeks, and that my prognosis for recovery was good. They also received clinical notes from Dr. King and Dr. Kennedy. They knew my date of birth, my employee number, even my union affiliation. But I didn't know Elizabeth's last name. She wouldn't extend me that courtesy.

The decision shocked the union and the CBC, both of whom called to demand a reversal. One week after I received the rejection letter, the company did exactly that. I was drafting an appeal letter when Elizabeth R. telephoned to say that the insurance company had changed its mind.

"I misinterpreted the contract," she said.

I was astonished, thankful, but still ticked. Elizabeth R. had managed to torque up the stress, needlessly.

Elizabeth said they don't reveal last names for security reasons. I did eventually find out what the R stands for. I've debated with myself about revealing it, but I'd feel terrible if a nut bar showed up on her doorstep. No, I'll keep it secret. Even though Elizabeth was always polite to me, Great-West Life's behaviour was mean-spirited, callous and indifferent. Collectively, they were rude. Let the R stand for that.

I went back to work February 25, 2008. There were innumerable handshakes and welcome backs.

I introduced myself to Christina Marshall, a young woman with a wide smile who joined the CBC during my sick leave and had replaced me on air.

"You had throat cancer, didn't you?" she asked.

"Yes, but I'm fine now."

There are no secrets in St. John's, especially inside the CBC. I had the impression that every time a doctor shoved a scope up my nose, the picture popped up on a television monitor inside the newsroom.

"Oh look, there's Glenn's throat. It's healing nicely. He'll be back to work soon."

I was on a graduated return to work program. Week one, I was expected to prepare one voice report, week two, two voice reports, and so on until week five, when I was supposed to be filing a report every day.

By week two, I was back to normal reporting duties. I had the energy to be on the air every day. Eventually, the producers thought my voice was strong enough to chance live hits into the show. My fear of dying a thousand deaths by having a coughing fit or cracking voice on televisions throughout Newfoundland and Labrador never materialized.

Cancer never seemed very far from me. One day, I was assigned to cover the inquiry into botched breast cancer tests. The scope of the mistakes had only widened since my last story on the subject. I thought again of my own misdiagnosis, and how lucky I was to have the mistake caught so quickly.

That March morning Patricia Goobie told the inquiry a heartbreaking story. Her sister, Geraldine Avery, had cancer in her right breast in 1999. It later spread to her other breast, to her chest and stomach. Because her test was read incorrectly, she was given tamoxifen almost six years too late. She died in 2006.

Ms. Goobie said, "Perhaps she would have died with cancer, we can't say that. But at least she would have been given a fair chance if she had been put on tamoxifen on the first of it in 1999. I don't think it would have come back in the second breast."

Watching her testify was the acting head of the Eastern Health Authority. I asked Louise Jones afterwards if she'd like to apologize to Ms. Goobie. She reacted incredulously.

"Sorry from me, what does it absolutely mean? These people have long-term relationships with their physicians, with their care providers. And there's lots to this story that we don't even know."

Louise Jones would eventually apologize profusely and sincerely for the health care system's failings. I never wanted an apology myself, and still don't. The pathologist who missed my cancer may have given me her best shot. The failing may have been in her training, or education. I really don't know. No one from the laboratory has ever talked to me about the error. I only hope that she's not missing somebody else's tonsil cancer.

By June it was clear that I was not going to put on any weight. My waistline had shrunk at least two inches, from a size 36 to a 34. If not for a belt, my pants would have dropped to my ankles. So I gathered up my entire summer wardrobe and went to the Vietnamese tailor downtown.

Kim Le wanted to pin the backside seam of each pair before taking them in. I was zipping in and out of the change room with abandon until I flung open the door, wearing shorts and socks, and stepped out in full view of the province's Minister of Natural Resources.

I had interviewed Kathy Dunderdale many times at the legislature, so she knew who I was.

"Hello, minister."

"Hello."

"Turn around," ordered Kim Le, and she proceeded to pin my ass in front of a Minister of the Crown.

I felt silly. Reporters and cabinet ministers will inevitably have prickly exchanges. I wondered, How will she keep a straight face the next time I have a go at her in a scrum?

All she had to do was think of that line from the musical *Les Miserables* to cut me down to size: "See them with their trousers off, they're never quite as grand."

"Boogers."

Dr. Lee was trying to manoeuvre the flexible scope up my left nostril and had run into a roadblock.

Mom used to say, "Always wear clean underwear. You never know when you're going to be in an accident." Had she been alive, she would probably have said, "Make sure your nose is clean. You never know when a doctor might want to stick a hose up there."

"Sorry," I said, a tad embarrassed. Dr. Lee had better luck with the right nostril.

"I've been having some pain in my ears," I said.

"Does the pain stay continuously or is it intermittent?"

"It comes and goes."

"That's good. Constant pain in an ear is a bad sign. It means the cancer might have come back."

Dr. Lee suspected that the pain was connected to the small ulcers that occasionally appeared in my throat, the consequence of a compromised immune system. The ulcers were caused by a virus and had to run their course.

Dr. Lee was about to give my neck its bimonthly groping when Dr. Norman walked into the examination room.

"Dr. Norman, you didn't call, you didn't write. I thought the relationship was over."

I didn't see Dr. Norman on my last visit to the cancer clinic. Dr. Lee was the lead doctor when it came to follow-up care, and Dr. Norman had moved on to other patients.

"Are you back to work yet?" she asked, ignoring my brilliant opening line.

"Dr. Norman, you're killing me. I've been back four months. That tells me you're not watching our newscast."

"I don't own a television, but if I did I'd watch CBC."

It was cold comfort. How was it possible that so many doctors and nurses, seemingly smart doctors and nurses, didn't watch *Here & Now?* The Evil Glenn figured that they actually did watch the show, but they wanted to make me squirm, just for the fun of it.

There was no point in ranting about medical indifference to my ego; it was show and tell time. I had something to show Dr. Lee — the answer to my question about how I could run with a dry mouth. The solution was a gift from Steve and Karen. They gave me an ingeniously designed water pouch. It was part of a belt that snapped around my waist and fit into the small of my back. A hose ran from the pouch underneath my arm and clipped onto my T-shirt, just below my chin. I could easily take a sip whenever I needed one. It made running possible. Steve and I were jogging three mornings a week around Kent's Pond. No hills and an easy trot for a couple of miles. I was back in the saddle, so to speak.

And there was an unexpected perk to my running again. Whenever I put the hose in my mouth, I looked like a Borg. There was still hope that Seven of Nine would give me a second look. Please, assimilate me.

I walked into Dr. Lee's office, pointed my two index fingers at him and said, "You, my friend, are getting a piece of caribou. It's hanging in the butcher's chill room right now."

"You got one?" There was surprise in his voice and on his face. "I just don't see you full of blood lust."

"To be honest, I don't see myself that way either. But for one week a year, it's like I'm a different person. I do feel a pang when I pull the trigger. But I think of the meat in the freezer and get on with it."

I promised Dr. Lee that I would attach a favourite recipe to the steak: caribou stew with porcini mushrooms served over gnocchi. I come by culinary adventures with caribou honestly. Fine food and drink are an integral part of each and every day in the Newfoundland wilderness. Steve and I might be killers, but we are not savages.

We headed to the Gaff Topsails plateau with six bottles of wine clinking in the back of the truck, which allowed us to have preposterous conversations.

"Steve, would you like the Italian pinot grigio or the Portuguese chardonnay tonight?"

"Let's have the chardonnay with the mushroom caps stuffed with escargot, and the French merlot with the chicken breasts coated in partridgeberry pate."

I'm not making this up. Years ago, I outlined a similar wine and food menu to a colleague at work. She was both impressed and cutting. "You're such food snobs. It's like Niles and Frasier go hunting."

The caribou in the chill room was the culmination of five days on an ATV, bouncing over logging roads and abandoned railway beds. The caribou were scarce. On some days, we didn't see any. I had a stag-only license, so the few does we did see could prance by with no cause for concern. We were down to our last day. Things were looking grim. The guy who rented us his cabin offered to lead us to a "secret" bog. Gerald is a part-time trapper and woodsman extraordinaire. We jumped at the chance.

"I know where they breeds," he boasted in the Newfoundland vernacular.

The bog was surrounded by thick alders, impenetrable unless you knew the right spot. Branches lashed our faces; ruts and rocks punished our derrieres. ATVs are not built for comfort over rough terrain. But one will put up with anything to avoid the night of long faces, anything to avoid explaining to our wives how we spent all that money and came home empty-handed.

The first time I went hunting Deb said, "Now, if you don't come back with an animal this will be a complete waste of time and money." Talk about pressure. What did wives say to their husbands when families could actually starve to death if the Great White Hunter wasn't great?

The bog was beautiful. Splashes of red and orange shrubs, golden grass swaying like wheat, and a horizon that seemed like a day's walk away. When I squinted, I saw three caribou at the far end.

I took off my rain jacket and strapped on my water pouch. I took a sip from the hose. I was a Borg all right. I had a weapon, prey and no emotion.

It was surprisingly warm for a November day. We started walking. It took forever to reach the caribou. I peered through the binoculars. Two does and a stag. The stag was missing an antler, but that was immaterial. I'm not a trophy hunter.

We were hidden in a clump of trees. The stag was about 200 metres away, grazing on lichen. I couldn't sit or lie down. I would have to take the shot standing up, the worst possible position. I rested the barrel on a branch, slowed my breathing and pulled the trigger. My shot rang out at the 11th hour, but I made it count. The caribou reared up on its hind legs and dropped.

Caribou hunting is a bloody bit of business, quite apart from the killing. A caribou should be cleaned and quartered before it's moved to get the best quality meat. You can be up to your elbows in blood and guts in no time.

"Who's got the axe?" asked Gerald.

"Steve's got a saw, if you want," I said. The saw took more time, but was much neater.

"Ya, some fellas like the saw," said Gerald. The tone in his voice told us that he wasn't one of them. Steve dug out the axe from his knapsack. Gerald hacked his way through the chest bone with three or four good swings, and opened up the cavity.

I had a cold chill go through me. I suddenly had an image of me lying comatose on the operating room table and Dr. Lee asking, "Who's got the axe?"

When the job was done, we all toasted the caribou with a shot of straight rum. It burned my throat. One year after finishing radiation and I still couldn't tolerate hard liquor.

I called Deb's dad on my cell phone.

"Jim, this is your favourite son-in-law."

"You're not my favourite son-in-law unless you're bringing home steaks for my barbeque."

"Don't worry, the children won't starve this winter."

Steve and I split the caribou, and we both delivered food hampers to members of the family. I also gave caribou steak to three doctors. I wanted to do something personal to thank them for their professionalism and kindness.

My mother had told me that my grandfather's poorer patients often paid him with fish or vegetables. By offering my doctors caribou steak, I was keeping a Newfoundland tradition alive.

I plopped myself down in Sarah's dental chair for my final saliva test, the fourth since finishing radiation treatment.

"Swallow and open wide."

Sarah was using the same litmus paper test under my tongue that Dr. Maxymiw used in Toronto. After three minutes, the blue dye revealed that I had produced just 7 millimetres of saliva. A person with healthy salivary glands can produce 35 millimetres. I was terribly disappointed.

I had convinced myself that I was actually doing better. I occasionally interrupted dinner conversation to excitedly announce to Deb that I was swallowing something with no water.

"Here comes the daily saliva report," Deb would say, rolling her eyes.

Unfortunately, the last test was consistent with earlier tests. There was only miniscule improvement. There was no doubt; I had radiation-induced xerostomia — dry mouth. I was producing only one-fifth the normal flow of saliva. It had been a year since my return home. Many experts think that what you have after a year is what you'll have for the rest of your life. Guess I'd better get used to carrying a water bottle.

January 22, 2009: it was my fifty-first birthday and we were in New Yawk, baby.

Deb let me be boss for the day. I had complete control of the itinerary. We started with a boat ride to circumnavigate Manhattan, though it turned out to be more of a horseshoe excursion around Manhattan. We couldn't make the full circle because of "icebergs" at the northern tip of the island. I resisted the urge to explain the difference between ice pans and icebergs to the lady selling the tickets. No sense being an insufferable know-it-all on my birthday. There were lots of other days for that. I soaked up the views, ate a New York pretzel and was completely relaxed until I saw a couple from Victoria, British Columbia, whom we had met the day before.

We had all been ice-skating at the Rockefeller Center. I have to confess that we were a little smug about our skating ability. Bodies, presumably non-Canadian, were sprawling everywhere. It was a full-time job avoiding collisions.

And there they were, on the same tour boat as us, a day later. What were the odds? I jokingly accused them of stalking us, though I told Deb in private, "If I see them at the Empire State Building, I'm calling the cops."

We passed underneath the Brooklyn Bridge and I suggested to Deb that we walk it the next day. A look of dread came over her face. You'd think that I had suggested walking over a rope bridge in the Peruvian jungle.

"It is safe?" she asked innocently.

"Not really," the Evil Glenn said. "Cars fall through the bridge every day. Haven't you seen it on the news?"

"I wish they had irradiated your attitude."

After the boat ride we wandered around Times Square, and then caught a train to Chinatown. I struck up a conversation with a guy in a Chinese bakery (Deb has a weakness for egg tarts) who gave us directions to a street lined with Vietnamese restaurants. We strolled back and forth, and chose Nha Trang One. According to the poster in the window, the *New York Times* food critic loved it, and that was good enough for me. I knew we had picked the right spot after tasting the shrimp paste wrapped around sugarcane. We gorged ourselves on plates of frogs' legs with lemon grass and chilli, ginger chicken, and salted shrimp. Thank God, I discovered Vietnamese food at a young age.

We rolled out of the restaurant and headed for the Empire State Building. No line-up, so we zipped to the top. No sign of King Kong or the couple from Victoria, so it was safe to step out on the observation deck. What a gorgeous city! It was bloody cold eighty-six stories up, but the view was worth every shiver.

I was feeling genki. I thought of my doctors and smiled.

"You bastards did this to me," I said softly. "Thank you."

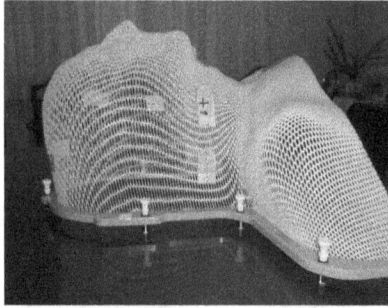

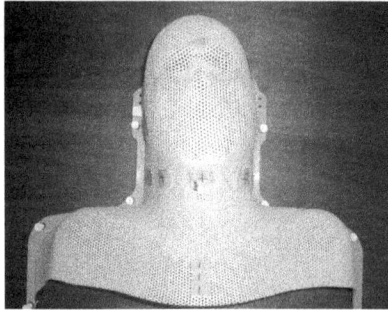

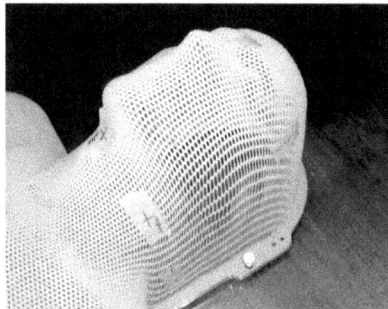

This is Glenn Deir's immobilization mask, the mask that pegged him to a table during his radiation treatment. He wore it 25 times over five weeks, approximately 15 to 20 minutes each time. In the final days of his treatment, he would occasionally fall asleep while wearing it.

Acknowledgments

In the early days of writing this book I didn't know whether I had written anything worth reading. I gave the first three chapters to my friend and former boss, Ron Crocker, and asked him to give me a brutally honest assessment. Our years together in CBC newsrooms in St. John's and Halifax had taught me that if the manuscript deserved to be torched, Ron would strike the match. To my great relief, he insisted that I finish it. Over the next year he provided countless sensible suggestions, unwavering encouragement, and the occasional recommendation to spike certain paragraphs. Thank you.

Thank you, as well, to three other early readers — Fred Greening, Derek Yetman and Mary Jane Webber. All three know me well enough to metaphorically slap me up the side of the head when I needed slapping. They were incredibly generous with their time. I'm in your debt.

All my early reviewers found an embarrassingly high number of missing words, spelling mistakes and misplaced commas. Fred — Mr. Grammar — has quite the knack for it. I give you fair warning. If Fred Greening says you need a comma, you need a comma. Question the suggestion and you run the risk of getting a lecture on the difference between coordinate and non-coordinate adjectives.

Even though I make my living as a television journalist, and occasionally get recognized on the street because of my job, in the publishing world I'm Glenn Who. Breakwater Books, and in particular managing editor Annamarie Beckel, has taken a chance on an unknown writer. I'm grateful.

The book contains previously unpublished material, except for portions of the story concerning Corporal Jamie Murphy and his family. Excerpts were taken from an article I wrote in the spring 2004 edition of *Media* magazine. They are reprinted with the editor's permission.

I owe a thousand thank yous for a thousand acts of kindness from friends and family members during and after radiation treatment. From shovelling the driveway, to writing funny notes, to cooking gentle food. I'm not the sentimental type, but you'll never know how much your actions meant to me.

Domo arigato gozaimashita.

www.ingramcontent.com/pod-product-compliance
Lightning Source LLC
Chambersburg PA
CBHW062224270326
41930CB00009B/1864